PUBLIC HEALTH IN THE 21ST CENTURY

DIETARY SUPPLEMENTS AND FDA USE OF ADVERSE EVENT REPORTS

PUBLIC HEALTH IN THE 21ST CENTURY

Additional books in this series can be found on Nova's website
under the Series tab.

Additional E-books in this series can be found on Nova's website
under the E-book tab.

NUTRITION AND DIET RESEARCH PROGRESS

Additional books in this series can be found on Nova's website
under the Series tab.

Additional E-books in this series can be found on Nova's website
under the E-book tab.

PUBLIC HEALTH IN THE 21ST CENTURY

DIETARY SUPPLEMENTS AND FDA USE OF ADVERSE EVENT REPORTS

WILLIAM M. FORSBERG
EDITOR

New York

For permission to use material from this book please contact us:
Telephone 631-231-7269; Fax 631-231-8175
Web Site: http://www.novapublishers.com

Library of Congress Cataloging-in-Publication Data

ISBN: 978-1-62808-023-0

Published by Nova Science Publishers, Inc. † New York

CONTENTS

PREFACE

Manufacturers, packers, and distributors of dietary supplements in the United States are required to report information about serious adverse effects associated with the use of these supplements to the Food and Drug Administration (FDA). The FDA carefully considers all the available safety information submitted to the agency before a product is approved. However, unexpected and sometimes serious safety problems can emerge once a product goes to market and is used by millions of people. As a result, postmarket safety monitoring, that is, analyzing information on products once they go to market, is a critical part of the FDA's responsibilities. The public provides an important source of such safety information. Health care facilities, practitioners, and patients submit reports to the FDA and to manufacturers on advise events, medical errors, and product quality problems observed during the use of a product. This book examines the number of adverse event reports the FDA has received since 2008; their source and types of products identified, and the actions the FDA has taken to ensure that firms are complying with adverse event report requirements.

Chapter 1 - Dietary supplements, such as vitamins and botanical products, are a multibillion dollar industry; national data show that over half of all U.S. adults consume them. FDA regulates dietary supplements and generally relies on postmarket surveillance, such as monitoring AERs, to identify potential concerns. Since December 2007, firms receiving a serious AER have had to report on it to FDA within 15 days. In January 2009, GAO reported that FDA had taken several steps to implement AER requirements and had recommended actions to help FDA identify and act on safety concerns for dietary supplements. GAO was asked to examine FDA's use of AERs in overseeing dietary supplements. This report examines the (1) number of AERs

FDA has received since 2008, their source, and types of products identified; (2) actions FDA has taken to ensure that firms are complying with AER requirements; (3) extent to which FDA is using AERs to initiate and support its consumer protection efforts; and (4) extent to which FDA has implemented GAO's 2009 recommendations. GAO analyzed FDA data, reviewed FDA guidance, and interviewed FDA officials.

Chapter 2 - Manufacturers, packers, and distributors of dietary supplements in the United States are required to report information about serious adverse effects associated with the use of these supplements to the Food and Drug Administration (FDA).

This requirement is detailed in the Dietary Supplement and Nonprescription Drug Consumer Protection Act, enacted on December 22, 2006. The effective date for complying with this requirement was December 22, 2007.

Chapter 3 - Contains questions and answers on dietary supplements from a U.S. Food and Drug Administration publication.

Chapter 4 - The FDA carefully considers all the available safety information submitted to the agency before a product is approved. However, unexpected and sometimes serious safety problems can emerge once a product goes to market and is used by millions of people.

As a result, postmarket safety monitoring, that is, analyzing information on products once they go to market, is a critical part of the FDA's responsibilities.

The public provides an important source of such safety information. Health care facilities, practitioners, and patients submit reports to the FDA and to manufacturers on adverse events, medical errors, and product quality problems observed during the use of a product. Reporting by facilities, practitioners and patients to the FDA or to manufacturers – known either as voluntary reporting when involving medical devices and spontaneous reporting when involving drugs and biologic products – is entirely voluntary and has increased greatly in recent years. In addition to voluntary reporting, there is mandatory reporting. Manufacturers who receive a report must submit it to the FDA and healthcare facilities must file reports of deaths and serious injuries involving medical devices.

In: Dietary Supplements and FDA Use … ISBN: 978-1-62808-023-0
Editor: William M. Forsberg

Chapter 1

DIETARY SUPPLEMENTS: FDA MAY HAVE OPPORTUNITIES TO EXPAND ITS USE OF REPORTED HEALTH PROBLEMS TO OVERSEE PRODUCTS*

United States Government Accountability Office

WHY GAO DID THIS STUDY

Dietary supplements, such as vitamins and botanical products, are a multibillion dollar industry; national data show that over half of all U.S. adults consume them. FDA regulates dietary supplements and generally relies on postmarket surveillance, such as monitoring AERs, to identify potential concerns. Since December 2007, firms receiving a serious AER have had to report on it to FDA within 15 days. In January 2009, GAO reported that FDA had taken several steps to implement AER requirements and had recommended actions to help FDA identify and act on safety concerns for dietary supplements. GAO was asked to examine FDA's use of AERs in overseeing dietary supplements. This report examines the (1) number of AERs FDA has received since 2008, their source, and types of products identified; (2) actions FDA has taken to ensure that firms are complying with AER

* This is an edited, reformatted and augmented version of the Highlights of GAO-13-244, a report to congressional requesters, dated March, 2013.

requirements; (3) extent to which FDA is using AERs to initiate and support its consumer protection efforts; and (4) extent to which FDA has implemented GAO's 2009 recommendations. GAO analyzed FDA data, reviewed FDA guidance, and interviewed FDA officials.

What GAO Recommends

GAO recommends, among other things, that FDA explore options to obtain poison center data, if determined to be useful; collect information on how it uses AERs; provide more information to the public about AERs; and establish a time frame to finalize guidance related to GAO's 2009 recommendations. FDA generally concurred with each of GAO's recommendations.

What GAO Found

From 2008 through 2011, the Department of Health and Human Services' Food and Drug Administration (FDA) received 6,307 reports of health problems—adverse event reports (AER)—for dietary supplements; 71 percent came from industry as serious adverse events as required by law, and most of these AERs were linked with supplements containing a combination of ingredients, such as vitamins and minerals or were otherwise not classified within FDA's product categories. However, FDA may not be receiving information on all adverse events because consumers and others may not be voluntarily reporting these events to FDA, although they may be contacting poison centers about some of these events. From 2008 to 2010, these centers received over 1,000 more reports of adverse events linked to dietary supplements than did FDA for the same period. FDA officials said that they are interested in determining whether the poison center data could be useful for their analysis and have held discussions with American Association of Poison Control Centers representatives, but cost is a factor.

To help ensure firms are complying with AER requirements (i.e., submitting serious AERs, maintaining AER records, and including firms' contact information on product labels), FDA increased its inspections of supplement firms and took some actions against noncompliant firms. Specifically, FDA increased firm inspections from 120 in 2008 to 410 from

January 1 to September 30, 2012. Over this period, FDA took the following actions: 3 warning letters, 1 injunction, and 15 import refusals related to AER violations, such as not including contact information on the product label or submitting a serious AER.

FDA has used AERs for some consumer protection actions (e.g., inspections and warning letters) but may be able to expand their use. FDA officials said that most AERs do not initiate or support such actions because it is difficult to establish causality between the product and the health problem based on the limited information in an AER. However, FDA does not systematically collect information on how it uses AERs for consumer protection actions; by collecting this information, it may be able to assess whether AERs are being used to their fullest extent. In addition, FDA is not required to provide information to the public about potential safety concerns from supplement AERs as it does for drugs. Making such information public, if consistent with disclosure provisions in existing law, could expand FDA's use of AERs and improve consumer awareness and understanding of potential health events associated with dietary supplements.

FDA has partially implemented all of GAO's 2009 recommendations, such as issuing guidance for new dietary ingredients, clarifying the boundary between dietary supplements and conventional foods, and expanding partnerships to improve consumer understanding. Specifically, FDA developed draft guidance in 2009, 2011, and 2012 to address three GAO recommendations about dietary supplement oversight and formed new partnerships to conduct consumer outreach. However, FDA has not issued final guidance in two cases. FDA officials said that they plan to complete implementation, but they have provided no time frame to do so. With final guidance in place, firms may be able to make more informed product development and marketing decisions, which could ultimately reduce FDA's enforcement burden in these areas.

ABBREVIATIONS

AAPCC	American Association of Poison Control Centers
AER	adverse event report
CAERS	CFSAN Adverse Event Reporting System
CDC	Centers for Disease Control and Prevention
CGMP	Current Good Manufacturing Practices
CFSAN	Center for Food Safety and Applied Nutrition

DSHEA	Dietary Supplement Health and Education Act
FDA	Food and Drug Administration
FSMA	FDA Food Safety Modernization Act of 2011
GRAS	generally recognized as safe
HHS	Department of Health and Human Services
NDI	New Dietary Ingredient
OEI	Official Establishment Inventory
RSS	Really Simple Syndication

March 18, 2013

The Honorable Henry A. Waxman
Ranking Member
Committee on Energy and Commerce
House of Representatives

The Honorable Richard J. Durbin
United States Senate

From 2009 to 2010, almost half of all U.S. adults consumed dietary supplements—including vitamins, minerals, and herbals—according to the Centers for Disease Control and Prevention, and dietary supplement sales surpassed $30 billion in 2011.[1] Furthermore, the number of supplements on the market has grown exponentially, from an estimated 4,000 products in 1994[2] to an estimated 55,000 products in 2009, according to officials from the U.S. Department of Health and Human Services' (HHS) Food and Drug Administration (FDA). In some cases, these products have caused serious health effects, as in the case of botanical ephedrine alkaloids—an herbal ingredient used in weight loss supplements that was linked to several deaths and banned from the dietary supplement market in 2004 and about which we reported in July 2003.[3]

FDA regulates dietary supplements under the Federal Food, Drug, and Cosmetic Act, as amended by the Dietary Supplement Health and Education Act of 1994 (DSHEA). Under DSHEA, FDA regulates dietary supplements, including vitamins, minerals, herbals and other botanicals, amino acids, certain other dietary substances, and derivatives of these items. DSHEA directs FDA to require in regulation that dietary supplement labels include a list of ingredients present in significant amounts and the quantity of such ingredients in the product.[4] Also, under DSHEA, FDA does not have the authority to require dietary supplements to be approved for safety and effectiveness before they enter the market, as it does for prescription drugs.[5] To identify potential safety concerns related to dietary supplements, FDA primarily relies on postmarket surveillance efforts, such as monitoring reports of health problems or adverse event reports (AER) it receives from industry, health care practitioners, and individuals; reviewing consumer complaints; and conducting inspections of dietary supplement firms. Once FDA identifies a safety concern, it may take an advisory action—such as sending a warning letter to a firm that manufactures, distributes, or packs a dietary supplement—or a regulatory action, including refusing entry to an imported product, seeking an injunction in federal court against a firm, or initiating a prosecution of a firm. FDA may also ban an ingredient through the rule-making process, as it did for botanical ephedrine alkaloids. If FDA decides to remove a product from the market using a regulatory action, it must demonstrate that the dietary supplement presents a significant or unreasonable risk of illness or injury[6] or is otherwise adulterated before it can do so. Collectively, in this report, we are referring to FDA's surveillance, advisory, and regulatory actions as consumer protection actions.

Since botanical ephedrine alkaloids were banned from dietary supplements in 2004, two major regulatory changes have occurred to address the oversight of dietary supplements. First, since December 2007, the Federal Food, Drug, and Cosmetic Act, as amended by the 2006 Dietary Supplement and Nonprescription Drug Consumer Protection Act (the 2006 act), has required dietary supplement manufacturers, distributors, or packers (dietary supplement firms) with their names appearing on the supplement label to report information about any serious AERs they receive to FDA within 15 business days of receiving the AER.[7] As defined in the act, serious adverse events include any health-related events that result in, for example, a death, life-threatening experience, inpatient hospitalization, or birth defect, or that require, based on reasonable medical judgment, a medical or surgical intervention to prevent these serious outcomes. The act does not require firms to report moderate or mild adverse events, such as gastrointestinal distress or headaches, but firms may do so voluntarily. Under the act, firms are also required to maintain records on each report of an adverse event (i.e., serious, moderate, and mild) for 6 years and allow HHS officials access to these records during an inspection or other limited circumstances, and firms must include a domestic address or domestic phone number on the dietary supplement product label for individuals to submit AERs. According to a report by the Senate Committee on Health, Education, Labor, and Pensions on the act, these AER requirements are intended to enhance FDA's ability to identify and act on public health issues associated with the use of dietary supplements.[8] Second, FDA established Current Good Manufacturing Practice (CGMP) regulations describing the conditions under which supplements must be manufactured, packed, and held. These requirements were implemented in phases, according to company size, and became fully effective in 2010.

In January 2009, we reported that FDA had taken several steps in response to the new mandatory AER requirements,[9] and we made the following four recommendations to enhance FDA's oversight of dietary supplements with which HHS generally agreed:

- FDA should request additional authority to (1) require dietary supplement firms to self-identify as dietary supplement firms and provide information on the products they sell annually as part of the existing process for firm registration and (2) require firms to report all mild and moderate adverse events to FDA. This recommendation addressed our finding that FDA's ability to identify safety concerns was hindered by a lack of information in three key areas: the identity and location of dietary supplement firms; the types and contents of products on the market; and product safety information, such as adverse event data.
- FDA should issue new dietary ingredient guidance clarifying when an ingredient is considered a new dietary ingredient, the evidence needed to document the safety of new dietary ingredients, and appropriate methods for establishing ingredient identity. This recommendation addressed our finding that FDA recognized the need to develop guidance on the new dietary ingredient provisions of DSHEA, but FDA had yet to issue this guidance—an omission previously highlighted in a report we issued in 2000.[10]
- FDA should issue guidance to industry clarifying when products should be marketed as dietary supplements or conventional foods formulated with added dietary ingredients.[11] This recommendation addressed our finding that the boundary between dietary supplements and foods containing added dietary ingredients, such as a beverage with kava, was not always clear.
- FDA should coordinate with stakeholder groups involved in consumer outreach to identify, implement, and assess the effectiveness of additional mechanisms for educating consumers about dietary supplements. This recommendation addressed our finding that

consumers remained largely uninformed about the safety, efficacy, and labeling of dietary supplements and that FDA could leverage its limited consumer outreach resources through partnerships with stakeholder groups.

You asked us to report on FDA's use of AERs in overseeing dietary supplements. We examined the (1) number of AERs FDA has received since 2008, the source of these reports, and the types of products identified; (2) actions FDA has taken to help ensure that firms are complying with the 2006 act's AER requirements; (3) extent to which FDA is using AERs to initiate and support its consumer protection actions; and (4) extent to which FDA has implemented our 2009 recommendations for enhancing FDA oversight of dietary supplements.

For this report, dietary supplement refers to a product intended for human consumption as defined in DSHEA—products that, among other things, are intended for ingestion to supplement the diet, labeled as a dietary supplement and not represented as a conventional food or as a sole item of a meal or diet. They must also contain one or more dietary ingredients. We did not examine FDA's oversight of products that would otherwise meet the definition of a dietary supplement in DSHEA but are intended for veterinary use. We also did not examine FDA's oversight of products that would otherwise meet the definition of a dietary supplement in DSHEA but are available only by prescription. We did include products that are marketed as dietary supplements but have been deliberately adulterated (e.g., tainted with active ingredients in FDA-approved drugs or their analogues to increase their potency). Although such products may not meet the legal definition of a dietary supplement because they contain prescription drug ingredients, we included them in our review because these products are often marketed as dietary supplements and can cause serious health problems. To identify how many AERs FDA has received since 2008, and the types of problems reported, we obtained and analyzed FDA data on the number and type of AERs received from January 2008 through December 2011. We supplemented our initial analysis with updated data on the number of AERs FDA received between January 1 and September 30, 2012. To assess the reliability of these data, we reviewed related documentation, examined data to identify obvious errors or inconsistencies, and worked with agency officials to identify any data problems. We determined the data to be sufficiently reliable for the purposes of this report. To examine FDA's actions to help ensure that firms are complying with the new reporting requirements, we reviewed the 2006 act, as well as FDA's procedures, planning documents, and guidance and obtained and analyzed data on FDA's oversight actions, such as inspections and regulatory activities, to identify which of these actions were related to monitoring or enforcing firms' compliance. To examine the extent to which FDA is using AERs for its consumer protection efforts, we used statistical software to match firm and product names from serious AERs against firm and product names from other FDA consumer protection actions from January 1, 2008, through December 31, 2011, such as inspections and warning letters, to identify which FDA actions were associated with a serious AER. We established a threshold for matching that gave us confidence we were capturing most of the potential matches and excluding those that were definitely not a match. The matches were then manually reviewed to confirm or reject potential matches. We verified the appropriateness of this approach with FDA officials. To determine the extent to which FDA has implemented GAO's 2009 recommendations for enhancing FDA oversight of dietary supplements, we reviewed relevant laws, planning documents, and guidance. We also reviewed proposed legislation to expand FDA's oversight authority for dietary supplements. In addition, to address all of our objectives, we reviewed relevant studies related to dietary supplements, adverse event reporting, industry compliance, and using poison center data for public health surveillance, among others. We reviewed the methodology for each of these studies and assessed them for reasonableness in accordance with our objectives. We interviewed officials from FDA's Center for Food Safety and Applied Nutrition (CFSAN) who receive and analyze AERs, officials from FDA's Division of Dietary Supplement Programs, officials from FDA's Office of Regulatory Affairs familiar with the agency's field operations and regulatory actions, and officials from FDA's Center for Drug Evaluation and Research. We also interviewed a wide range of stakeholders, including officials from HHS' Centers for Disease Control and Prevention and National Institutes of Health; and representatives of industry and trade organizations, consumer advocacy groups, and the American Association of Poison Control Centers. A more detailed description of our objectives, scope, and methodology is presented in appendix I.

We conducted this performance audit from December 2011 to March 2013 in accordance with generally accepted government auditing standards. Those standards require that we plan and perform the audit to obtain sufficient, appropriate evidence to provide a reasonable basis for our findings and conclusions based on our audit objectives. We believe that the evidence obtained provides a reasonable basis for our findings and conclusions based on our audit objectives.

Background

Responsibility for dietary supplement oversight is shared among several offices at FDA:

- FDA's Center for Food Safety and Applied Nutrition (CFSAN) manages the CFSAN Adverse Event Reporting System (CAERS), which collects and stores AERs related to foods and dietary supplements.[12] CFSAN also houses the Division of Dietary Supplement Programs, within its Office of Nutrition, Labeling and Dietary Supplements, which is responsible for developing guidance, providing scientific and technical expertise, and directing dietary supplement priorities across the agency. Additionally, CFSAN's Office of Compliance has primary responsibility for compliance and enforcement of FDA regulations and federal laws within FDA's jurisdiction with respect to foods—such as dietary supplements—including coordinating compliance and regulatory actions within the center and with other FDA components.[13] Among other responsibilities, the Office of Compliance reviews incoming investigational findings and recommendations to determine if a proposed action or remedy is supported by the documented observations and other evidence; assesses the integrity and relevance of the evidence; and obtains necessary scientific verification from appropriate subject matter experts.

FDA's Office of Regulatory Affairs is responsible for managing the agency's field operations in 25 regional and district offices for each of FDA's centers, including CFSAN. Among other responsibilities, the Office of Regulatory Affairs supports FDA centers by performing inspections and import operations. The Office of Regulatory Affairs also takes advisory and regulatory actions for dietary supplements, but generally these actions are coordinated with CFSAN's Office of Compliance.[14]

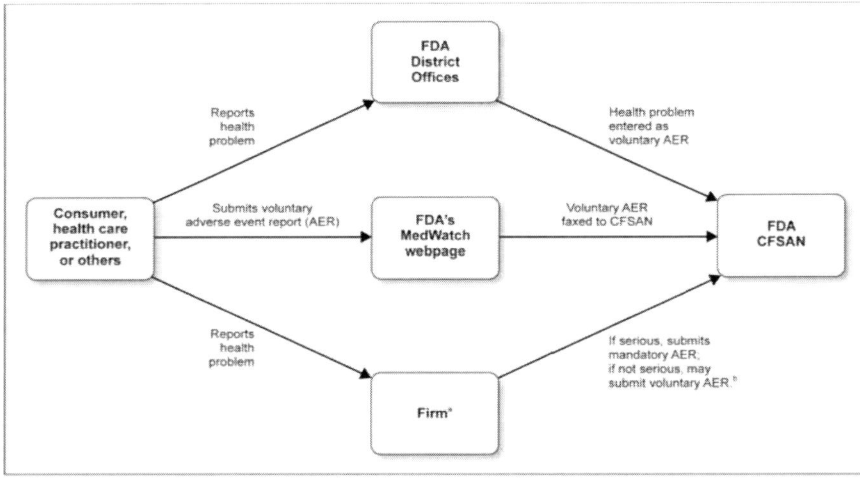

Source: GAO.

[a] Dietary supplement manufacturer, packer, or distributor identified on product label as the contact for AERs.

[b] As defined by the Federal Food, Drug, and Cosmetic Act, as amended by the 2006 act, serious adverse events include any health-related events that result in, for example, a death, life-threatening experience, inpatient hospitalization, or birth defect or that require, based on reasonable medical judgment, a medical or surgical intervention to prevent these serious outcomes. As provided in the 2006 act, the manufacturer, packer, or distributor of a dietary supplement with their name appearing on the label of a dietary supplement marketed in the United States, shall submit to the Secretary of HHS any report received of a serious adverse event associated with such dietary supplement when used in the United States, accompanied by a copy of the label on or within the retail packaging of such dietary supplement. The 2006 act does not require firms to report moderate or mild adverse events, such as gastrointestinal distress or headaches, but firms may do so voluntarily.

Figure 1. Process for Reporting a Health Problem as an Adverse Event for Dietary Supplements.

- FDA's Center for Drug Evaluation and Research is responsible for oversight of over-the-counter and prescription drugs, including generic drugs and some biological therapeutics. Center for Drug Evaluation and Research officials work with other FDA offices to identify products that are marketed as dietary supplements but that have been deliberately adulterated with active ingredients in FDA-approved drugs or their analogues. Once identified, FDA alerts the public and takes action to protect the public through a variety of consumer protection actions, such as working with firms on voluntary product recalls. Table 2 provides examples of consumer protection actions FDA may take in response to identified safety concerns.

According to FDA officials, the estimated resources for all dietary supplement activities across FDA grew slightly from $14.6 million in fiscal year 2009 to a projected $18.9 million in fiscal year 2012. These activities include regulatory and technical review, policy and guidance development, research, education and outreach, compliance and inspection activities, and associated administrative support activities, including infrastructure costs.

There are three different paths consumers, health care practitioners, or others can follow for reporting any serious, moderate, or mild health problem related to a dietary supplement to FDA. First, consumers, health care practitioners, or others can complete an electronic voluntary AER form at FDA's MedWatch webpage—FDA's agencywide safety information and adverse event reporting program—and submit it to FDA. The information is then sent to CFSAN via fax.[15] Second, consumers, health care practitioners, or others can report the health problem to the dietary supplement firm listed on the product label. The firm evaluates the problem and, if it determines it to be serious in accordance with the 2006 act, it is to complete a hard copy mandatory AER form and submit the form to FDA by mail, along with a copy of the product label. If the firm determines the problem is not serious, it can complete and submit a voluntary AER form at its discretion. Third, consumers, health care practitioners, or others can report the health problem to an FDA Consumer Complaint Coordinator. The coordinators are located in FDA district offices and document and follow up on a variety of health and nonhealth-related complaints about FDA-regulated products.

Coordinators enter health problems reported by consumers into a database from which the health problems are later uploaded into the CAERS database as voluntary AERs, as shown in figure 1.[16]

Alternatively, consumers, health care practitioners, or others can call a poison center about a health problem.[17] Poison centers are independently operated and provide free medical advice from health care professionals who are trained in the toxicological management of poison exposures and can address toxic exposure situations and adverse events.[18] Poison exposures can result from a variety of circumstances and substances, including adverse reactions to dietary supplements under use as directed.[19] Calls received at the 57 poison centers covering the United States and its territories are uploaded into a national database for analysis. However, the 57 poison centers are not an adverse event reporting system. Consequently, individual health problems involving dietary supplements and managed as poison exposure cases by poison centers are generally not sent to CFSAN.[20]

When reporting a health problem to FDA, individuals are asked to provide a short description of the reported health problem; a brief description of the affected person, such as age, gender, weight, and any preexisting medical conditions; and information about the dietary supplement, such as the product name and manufacturer, as well as dosage associated with the health problem. Firms submitting mandatory AERs are also asked to provide the above information. However, to avoid duplication in its database, FDA asks for the following five data elements at a minimum for mandatory AERs: (1) an identifiable patient, (2) an identifiable individual who is reporting the health problem to the firm, (3) identity and contact information for the responsible firm submitting the serious AER to FDA, (4) a suspect dietary supplement, and (5) a serious adverse event or fatal outcome.

Once FDA receives an AER for a serious, moderate, or mild health problem, contractors enter the information into the CAERS database, either electronically or manually, and record information by product, industry code, ingredient(s), medical symptom(s) and other information.[21] CAERS staff review the AERs for accuracy and then distribute them to subject matter experts within CFSAN's program offices, including the Division of Dietary Supplement Programs, for their review.[22] These subject matter experts review the AERs to determine the extent of the relationship between the reported health problem and the product. In addition, CAERS data analysts use statistical tools to analyze relationships across all AERs to detect potential indicators of unsafe products, including patterns or relationships among health problems, products, and ingredients that are found to be significant, according to CFSAN officials. These officials said that, if CFSAN's subject matter experts find that a product in an AER contains active ingredients in FDA-approved drugs or their analogues, the AER is shared with FDA's Center for

Drug Evaluation and Research, which shares oversight responsibility for supplement products that have been deliberately adulterated with active ingredients in FDA-approved drugs or their analogues. If an issue related to compliance with dietary supplement regulations is identified—such as CGMPs describing the conditions under which supplements must be manufactured, packed, and held—CFSAN's subject matter experts pass the AER or cluster of AERs to CFSAN's Office of Compliance, which works with FDA's Office of Regulatory Affairs to determine if consumer protection actions are needed, as shown in figure 2.

FDA uses other postmarket surveillance approaches in addition to AERs to identify potential safety concerns and conduct oversight related to dietary supplements. Examples of these approaches are listed in table 1.

Table 1. Examples of FDA Surveillance Actions in Addition to AERs

Type of action	Description
Consumer complaints	Consumers or other parties can contact FDA to submit complaints about FDA-regulated products by phone. Complaints may address any aspect of a product including, but not limited to, an adverse event. In one instance, a complaint indicated that the dropper dispenser in a liquid dietary supplement broke during use. In another instance, a fish oil dietary supplement had a rotten fish smell.
Import screening	FDA reviews imported dietary supplement products and ingredients entering the country. There were approximately 546,603 dietary supplement shipments entering the country from 2008 to 2011. A small percentage of these products is examined or sampled.[a]
Inspections	FDA inspects firms that manufacture, pack, or hold dietary supplements. There are four general types of inspections: routine surveillance, consumer complaint investigations, for-cause compliance inspections, and follow-up to a regulatory action. An inspection may include product examinations, sampling and testing, as well as the inspection of the firm and facility involved with dietary supplements, according to FDA officials.
Internet monitoring	FDA monitors the Internet to identify products that purport to be dietary supplements but may be fraudulently promoted as drugs for treating disease.

Source: GAO.

[a] We did not collect data on the percentage of dietary supplement import entries that FDA examined, sampled, or tested for this report. However, in our prior work on dietary supplements (GAO-09-250), we found that FDA sampled or examined, on average, approximately 3 to 5 percent of dietary supplement import entries from fiscal year 2002 through March 24, 2008. According to FDA, an import entry line is each portion of an import shipment that is listed as a separate item on an entry document. Items in an import entry having different tariff descriptions must be listed separately.

According to FDA officials, inspections of dietary supplement firms constitute the agency's primary method for monitoring compliance with requirements to report adverse events. According to CFSAN guidance, FDA investigators take several steps during inspections to monitor compliance with AER requirements, including determining whether a firm has a process in place to report serious adverse events, determining whether the firm has any serious AERs that it did not submit to FDA, and reviewing labels to determine if the product has contact information for reporting AERs.

As table 2 shows, once FDA has identified a potential safety concern or a violation for dietary supplements, it has a range of consumer protection actions available, from advisory actions, such as issuing a warning letter, to regulatory actions, such as seizing adulterated dietary supplements.

According to FDA officials, products or ingredients of greatest concern for public health are subject to regulatory actions. In addition, FDA may pursue a regulatory action against a firm if the firm does not correct violations in response to an advisory action, such as a warning letter.

FDA Received More than 6,000 AERs Over 4 Years, but Consumers and Others May Not be Voluntarily Reporting All Adverse Events to FDA

FDA received more than 6,000 AERs from 2008 through 2011, primarily from industry, and most of these AERs were for supplements containing a combination of different types of ingredients (e.g., vitamins and minerals) or supplements that were otherwise not classified into one of FDA's existing product categories, according to our analysis of FDA data. However, FDA may not have received information on all adverse events that are associated with dietary supplements because consumers and others may not be voluntarily reporting them to FDA—either directly or through firms—although they may be contacting poison centers about some of these events. Specifically, poison centers received over 1,000 more reports of adverse events from 2008 through 2010 than FDA did.

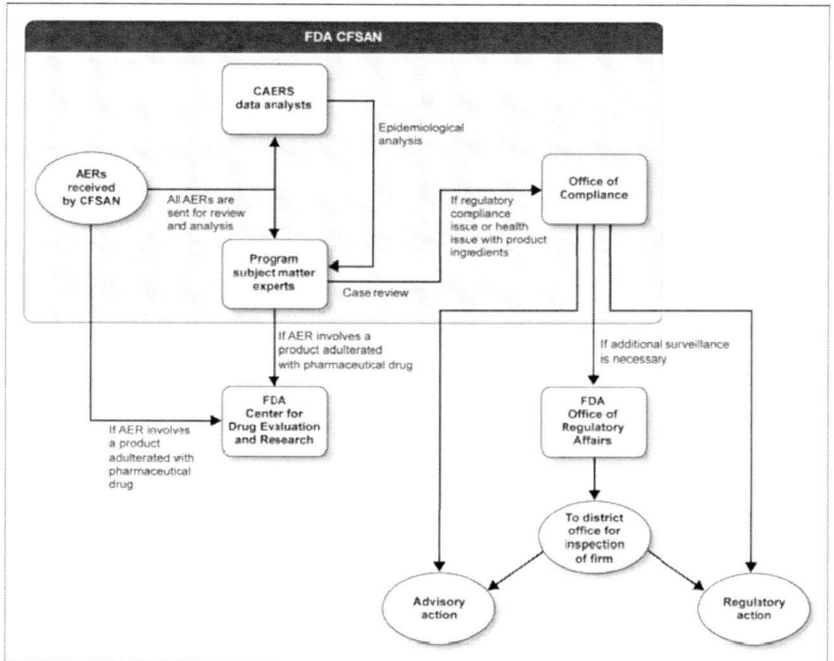

Source: GAO.

Note: Consumer complaints that involve health problems and are entered into CAERS as voluntary AERs, are sent directly to the Office of Compliance. Additionally, foreign inspections of firms are coordinated through the Office of Regulatory Affairs' headquarters, according to FDA officials.

Figure 2. Process for Reviewing AERs and Using AERs for Consumer Protection Actions.

Table 2. Examples of FDA Consumer Protection Actions in Response to Identified Potential Safety Concerns for Dietary Supplements

Type of action	Description
Advisory	
Warning letter	FDA issues a letter to a firm citing violations of statute or regulations. FDA may bring an enforcement action if a firm does not correct violations in response to a warning letter.
Consumer alert	FDA issues a public alert about types of products, ingredients, unlawful marketing practices, or other areas of concern.
Industry advisory	FDA issues an industrywide advisory urging firms not to market products containing certain ingredients or to address other areas of concern.
Regulatory	
Product recall	FDA works with firms to voluntarily remove a product from the market through a recall. According to FDA officials, the agency may also use its new mandatory recall authority for dietary supplement products when there is a reasonable probability that the dietary supplement is adulterated or misbranded because they contain a major food allergen. FDA received this authority in 2011 with the passage of the FDA Food Safety Modernization Act.[a]
Refusal of imported product	Imported products can be detained and subsequently refused entrance into the U.S. market at the port of entry.
Legal action	FDA can take legal action against firms, such as seeking seizures or injunctions, and the initiating of criminal charges against responsible parties.
Ban ingredient	FDA may issue a regulation banning an ingredient from the dietary supplement market.[b]

Source: GAO.

Note: This table is not an exhaustive list of potential consumer protection actions FDA could take. For example, FDA could hold a regulatory meeting with a firm to discuss voluntary action. However, we focused on these actions for the purposes of this report because (a) FDA maintained data on these actions or data were publicly available, or (b) we had reviewed these actions as part of our prior work on FDA's oversight of dietary supplements, GAO-09-250 .

[a] In January 2011, the FDA Food Safety Modernization Act amended the Federal Food, Drug, and Cosmetic Act to give FDA authority to order the recall of food products (other than infant formula) that present a reasonable probability of being adulterated or misbranded, with regard to a major food allergen, when a company fails to voluntarily recall the products. FDA already had authority to order the recall of infant formula.

[b] To date, FDA has banned one ingredient—botanical ephedrine alkaloids—in 2004.

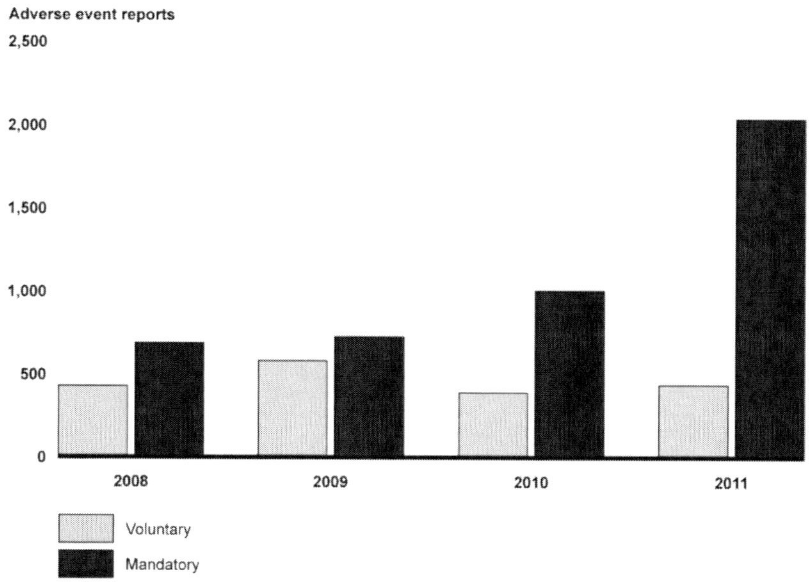

Source: GAO analysis of FDA data.

Note: In some cases, FDA received both voluntary and mandatory AERs for the same adverse event. To avoid double-counting, we included these cases in the mandatory AER total. FDA received from 12 to 24 AERs per year as both mandatory and voluntary from 2008 through 2011.

Figure 3. The Number of Voluntary and Mandatory Industry AERs Related to Dietary Supplements FDA Received, 2008 through 2011.

FDA Received 6,307 AERs from 2008 through 2011, Primarily from Industry, and Mostly for Combination Products or Unclassified Products

From 2008 through 2011, FDA received a total of 6,307 AERs related to dietary supplements; 71 percent of these AERs came from industry for serious health problems (i.e., based on consumer, health care practitioner, or others' reports), and most of these AERs were linked with dietary supplements containing a combination of ingredients—such as products containing both vitamins and minerals or otherwise unclassified dietary supplements—according to our analysis of FDA data. Specifically, the total number of AERs FDA received annually more than doubled over the period, from 1,119 in 2008 to 2,480 in 2011. This rise in AERs was driven by a large increase in the number of mandatory industry AERs, according to our analysis. As shown in figure 3, mandatory AERs almost tripled from 2008 through 2011, from 689 in 2008 to 2,040 in 2011. During the same period, AERs submitted voluntarily by consumers, industry, health care practitioners, and others remained relatively stable, averaging 461 annually.[23] All mandatory AERS from industry involved serious health problems, and FDA classified roughly 64 percent (1,179) of all voluntary AERs (1,844) as "serious as reported." "Serious as reported" means that the adverse event met the criteria to be classified as serious as it was reported to FDA (based on the reporter's responses to standard questions about it), whether or not FDA's later medical review classified it as serious. Appendix II incorporates data on AERs from our 2009 report to provide information on AERs FDA received from January 1, 2003, through September 30, 2012.[24]

According to FDA officials, two factors are driving the increase in mandatory AERs. First, FDA has increased its enforcement efforts against AER noncompliance. For example, FDA has taken advisory actions, such as issuing warning letters, against firms that have not reported serious AERs or failed to include contact information to report an adverse event on the product label. Second, lawsuits have publicized the consequences of adverse events and a firm's decision not to report these events. Specifically, a number of lawsuits have been filed against firms that produced and distributed Hydroxycut™—a weight loss supplement linked to serious liver damage—that cite FDA's request for a recall because of AERs as evidence.[25] In addition, in 2011, the Supreme Court ruled in favor of investors suing a publicly traded drug manufacturing firm for securities fraud, allowing shareholders to rely on the firm's decision not to report, among other things, AERs as grounds for a claim in their suit.[26] FDA officials stated that these lawsuits have raised firms' sensitivity to the risk involved in noncompliance with AER requirements, leading to the increase in mandatory AERs.

The 6,307 AERs FDA received from 2008 to 2011 reported the following serious outcomes:

- 53 percent (3,370) resulted in unspecified important medical events of a serious nature,
- 29 percent (1,836) resulted in hospitalization,
- 20 percent (1,272) resulted in serious injuries or illnesses,
- 8 percent (512) resulted in a life-threatening condition, and
- 2 percent (92) resulted in death.[27]

When interpreting AERs, FDA officials said that it is important to understand that an AER by itself does not demonstrate a causal relationship between the dietary supplement and the reported health problem.[28] Rather, the officials said that there are several other factors that must be considered to determine causality, such as the role of other products consumed at the same time and preexisting health conditions. Some demographic information on the individuals affected by these and other outcomes in the AERs was available. Specifically, of the 6,307 AERs, 63 percent (3,980) affected females; however, the age of the individual affected was missing in about one-third (2,029) of the AERs. According to FDA officials, the absence of such information can hinder the agency's ability to determine whether there is a causal relationship between the product and the reported health problem.

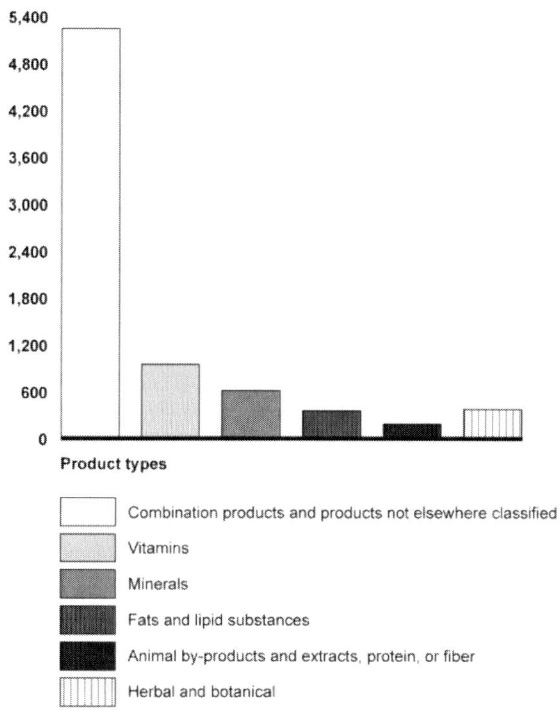

Source: GAO analysis of FDA data.

Note: Combination products included were a combination of different types of ingredients, such as vitamins and minerals.

Figure 4. Most Commonly Reported Types of Supplements Associated with Adverse Events, 2008 through 2011.

As shown in figure 4, the vast majority (5,248) of the supplements identified in the AERs were a combination of different types of dietary ingredients (e.g., vitamins and minerals) or supplements that were not otherwise classified by FDA into one of the agency's existing supplement categories. Vitamins were the second most frequently reported supplement, included in 952 AERs, followed by minerals, included in 619 AERs. According to FDA officials, the predominance of combination and unclassified supplements in AERs reflects the growing number of complex supplements on the market. These officials said that these supplements are challenging for FDA because of limited scientific knowledge on how different supplement ingredients interact and their effect on consumers' health. Although product names are not standardized within CAERs, we matched firm and product names across AERs data to estimate which types of products were associated with the most mandatory AERs.[29] According to our analysis, 6 of the 10 supplements receiving the most mandatory AERs were multivitamins; 2 were weight-loss supplements; 1 was an energy supplement, and 1 was an herbal concentrate. Three supplements were associated with over roughly 100 AERs; 7 were associated with about 51 to 100 AERs; and 24 were associated with about 26 to 50 AERs. Most of the supplements identified in the mandatory AERs were associated with approximately one AER from 2008 to 2011.[30]

Consumers and Others May Not be Voluntarily Reporting All Adverse Events to FDA, but May be Contacting Poison Centers about Some Events

FDA relies on consumers, health care practitioners, and others to voluntarily report adverse events associated with dietary supplements to FDA and to firms and, in turn, FDA relies on firms to submit to it any serious AERs it receives from these individuals, as required by law. However, FDA may not receive information on all adverse events that are associated with dietary supplements because consumers and others may not be voluntarily reporting these AERs—either directly or through firms, as indicated by our analysis and interviews with FDA officials. We found several potential reasons for this underreporting based on our review of relevant studies and our prior work. For example, we and others have reported that consumers, health care practitioners, or others may not recognize the chronic or cumulative toxic effects of a dietary supplement, or they may broadly assume dietary supplements to be safe and not attribute negative effects to them.[31] Additionally, in an October 2012 report, the HHS Office of Inspector General found that 20 percent of a judgmental sample of 127 weight loss and immune support dietary supplements did not have contact information that would enable consumers and health care practitioners to report adverse events.[32] The HHS Inspector General study is not representative of the dietary supplement industry but indicates that some firms may not be providing consumers with the necessary information to report adverse events to firms, which could lead to underreporting if consumers do not report the adverse event directly to FDA. FDA officials said that they receive fewer AERs than they would expect to given the number of dietary supplements on the market and their widespread use. However, they said that, similar to other voluntary reporting systems, the extent of underreporting is unknown because the agency can only know about those adverse events that are reported to it.[33]

One potential measure of underreporting is the number of dietary supplement-related health problems managed as poison exposure cases by poison centers. According to annual reports by the American Association of Poison Control Centers (AAPCC), poison centers received 145,775 calls from consumers or others related to dietary supplements from 2008 through 2010.[34] These include cases in which the consumer took more than the directed amount of a product, accidentally ingested the product, or used the product as directed but experienced an adverse event.[35] According to AAPCC reports, there were 4,863 cases of adverse events from 2008 to 2010, over 1,000 more than the 3,827 AERs FDA received during the same period.[36] We could not estimate how much overlap, if any, occurred between cases reported to FDA and the poison centers or determine whether some of the cases managed by poison centers were serious and might have also been reported to firms. However, the greater number of calls received by poison centers suggests that consumers, health care practitioners, and others may have contacted poison centers without reporting the adverse event to FDA.

FDA officials said that they are interested in reviewing the poison center data related to dietary supplements and have held discussions with AAPCC representatives. Specifically, CFSAN officials said that they want to review the raw poison center data on dietary supplements to understand what it includes and whether it would be useful for their analysis. However, these officials said that they were unable to review the raw dietary supplement data without purchasing it and said that FDA should have access to the data at no additional cost given the current level of federal support for poison centers.[37] For example, a 2012 study commissioned by the AAPCC, federal funding accounted for an estimated 13 percent (about $17 million) of poison centers' annual operating budget in 2011.[38] An FDA official noted that, in a 2004 report, the Institute of Medicine recommended that poison center data become available to all appropriate local, state, and federal public health units on a real-time basis and at no additional cost.[39] In this report, the Institute of Medicine also recommended that poison centers receive sufficient federal funding to cover core activities, which at the time were estimated to cost approximately $100 million annually.[40] According to AAPCC representatives, AAPCC does not receive federal appropriations to cover cost of collecting, maintaining, and sharing poison center data at the national level and generally charges federal agencies to access the data.[41]

AAPCC representatives also said that they were willing to work with FDA on reduced pricing. Specifically, based on a May 2012 quote, accessing 4 years' worth of AAPCC data of about 5,400 product codes would have cost almost $76 million prior to the AAPCC discount, and $800,000 after the discount. However, even with the significant AAPCC discount, access to the data remained more than twice the nearly $400,000 budgeted to process and perform surveillance of dietary supplement adverse events in fiscal year 2011.[42] According to CFSAN officials, as of October 2012, negotiations with AAPCC had stalled at the CFSAN level. CFSAN officials said that the cost of accessing the data was a factor. They also said that, although negotiations had stalled at the CFSAN level, as of December, 2012, they were ongoing at the department level, but from their perspective, progress remained difficult.

According to CFSAN officials, the greatest challenge for identifying potential safety concerns from AERs is the small number of AERs that FDA receives related to dietary supplements.[43] Specifically, these officials said that it is difficult to establish a baseline of doses and responses to help the agency detect anomalies that might indicate a potential safety concern using such a small number of AERs. These officials also said that they could not determine whether the poison center data would be useful for such signal detection until they could access it. However, researchers and the HHS Inspector General have concluded that accessing poison center data may help FDA detect and monitor potential safety concerns.[44] For example, a 2008 study performed in conjunction with CFSAN and the San Francisco Division of the California Poison Control System concluded that active surveillance of poison center reports of dietary supplement adverse events could enable rapid detection of potentially harmful products and may facilitate oversight.[45] Additionally, under contract with the AAPCC, the Centers for Disease Control and Prevention (CDC)—like FDA, an HHS component—has used national poison center data to identify and track adverse events related to dietary supplements. For example, in March 2008, poison centers in three states (Florida, Georgia, and Tennessee), state health departments, and FDA began receiving voluntary AERs of muscle cramps, hair loss, and joint pain related to Total Body Formula and Total Body Mega Formula. On FDA's behalf, CDC scientists used national poison center data to identify which states were reporting similar cases and to track the geographical extent of the outbreak.[46] If FDA can access more information about dietary supplement-related adverse events that are reported to poison centers, FDA may be able to analyze the increased data on doses and responses to help it identify potential safety concerns.

FDA Has Increased Its Compliance Monitoring of Firms and Taken Some Advisory and Regulatory Actions

To help ensure firms are complying with AER requirements for submitting serious AERs, maintaining AER records, and including AER contact information on supplement labels, from 2008 through 2011, FDA increased its monitoring of firms through inspections and has taken some advisory and regulatory actions against noncompliant firms.

FDA Has Increased its Monitoring of Firms through Inspections Since 2008

FDA has increased its compliance monitoring of firms through inspections to help ensure that dietary supplement firms are complying with AER requirements for (1) reporting serious AERs within 15 business days, (2) maintaining AER records for 6 years, and (3) including domestic contact information on product labels for individuals to submit AERs, according to our analysis of FDA data. Specifically, in 2008, FDA inspected 120 dietary supplement firms, which represented at least 6 percent of FDA's total inventory of dietary supplement firms at the beginning of 2008.[47] In contrast, from January through September 2012, FDA inspected 410 dietary supplement firms, which represented at least 18 percent of FDA's total inventory of dietary supplement firms at the beginning of 2012. FDA also increased the number of foreign firms it inspected over this period, from conducting no inspections in 2008 to conducting 35 from January through September 2012. Figure 5 shows the number of foreign and domestic inspections of dietary supplement firms FDA or its partners at the state level conducted annually from January 1, 2008 to September 30, 2012.[48]

According to FDA officials, the key factors underlying this increase in inspections were the full implementation of dietary supplement CGMP regulations in 2010 (i.e., describing the conditions under which supplements must be manufactured, packed, and held) and an increase in field investigators available to conduct inspections. The dietary supplement CGMP regulations established new quality control standards for dietary supplement firms and new compliance criteria for FDA investigators to use during dietary supplement inspections.

The CGMPs were phased in by firm size starting in 2008, with full implementation completed in 2010. Additionally, an FDA official said that new field investigators became available to conduct inspections in 2010 and 2011. These investigators had been hired following higher appropriations for FDA in fiscal years 2008 and 2009, but they did not become available to conduct inspections until 2010 and 2011 because it takes 1 to 2 years of training before an investigator is ready to perform inspections, according to this official.

As the CGMPs were being phased in, FDA identified problems or concerns during inspections, such as a manufacturer not maintaining, cleaning, or sanitizing equipment.[49] The percentage of inspections where FDA identified problems or concerns increased from 51 percent in 2008 to 73 percent in 2011, largely resulting from CGMP inspections, according to our analysis. See figure 6 for the proportion of dietary supplement inspections where FDA identified problems or concerns from 2008 to 2011.

According to our analysis of FDA inspection results from fiscal years 2008 through 2012, FDA identified 20 problems related to AER requirements during inspections.

In 3 of these instances, FDA found that the firm did not submit a mandatory AER within the required 15 days. In the 17 other instances, FDA found that a firm did not submit a mandatory AER. When FDA identifies a problem during an inspection, firms may decide to take voluntary corrective action, or FDA may choose to take an advisory or regulatory action against the firm for the observed violations.

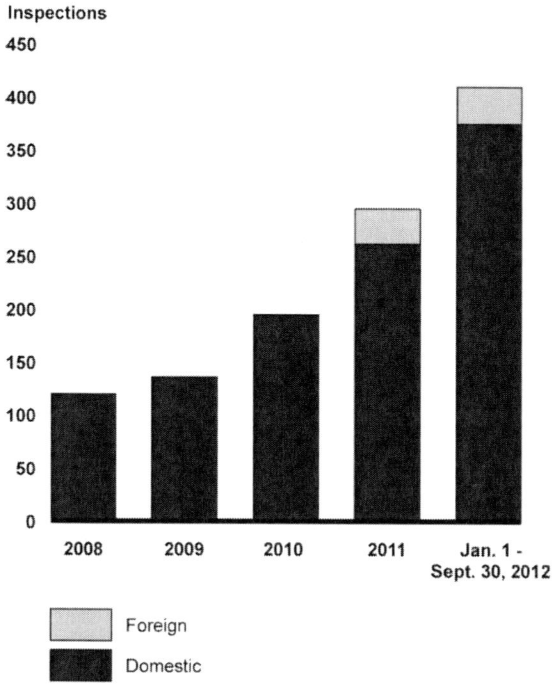

Source: GAO analysis of FDA data.

Note: FDA contracts with states to conduct domestic facility inspections for foods and other regulated products. During this period, states conducted 35 dietary supplement inspections on FDA's behalf.

Figure 5. Number of Foreign and Domestic Inspections of Dietary Supplement Firms FDA or Its State Partners Conducted, January 1, 2008 through September 30, 2012.

FDA Took a Total of 19 Advisory and Regulatory Actions Related to AER Noncompliance from January 2008 through December 2011

We identified a total of 19 advisory and regulatory actions that FDA initiated from 2008 to 2011 for noncompliance with AER requirements. Specifically, we found three warning letters (advisory actions), one injunction (regulatory action) to prevent the sale of a firm's products, and 15 import refusals (regulatory actions). All three of the warning letters stated that the supplement label did not include domestic contact information so that individuals could report an adverse event. The injunction against the dietary supplement manufacturer cited noncompliance with several sections of the Federal Food, Drug and Cosmetic Act, including the failure to report serious adverse events as required by law. It prohibited the firm from producing and distributing over 400 products; this was the first time FDA had taken legal action against a large manufacturer for CGMP noncompliance, according to FDA documents. All of the 15 import refusals—spanning nine supplement companies—that we identified cited violations of supplement labeling requirements for domestic contact information so that individuals can report an adverse event. Table 3 provides more information on the 19 advisory and regulatory actions related to noncompliance with AER requirements that we identified.

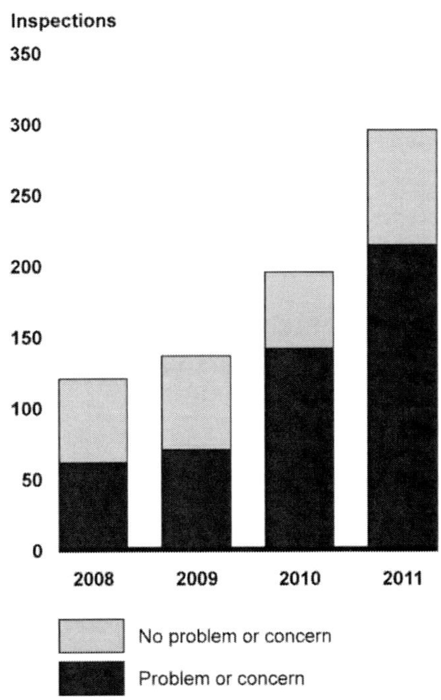

Source: GAO analysis of FDA data.

Note: Dietary supplement CGMPs were phased in by firm size from 2008 to 2010. For firms with 500 or more full-time equivalent employees, they became effective in June 2008; for firms with at least 20 but fewer than 500 full-time equivalent employees, they became effective in June 2009; and for firms with fewer than 20 full-time equivalent employees they became effective in June 2010.

Figure 6. Proportion of Dietary Supplement Inspections for Which FDA Identified Problems or Concerns, 2008 through 2011.

Table 3. Identified Advisory and Regulatory Actions on AER Requirement Violations, 2008 through 2011

Initiation date[a]	Action date	Firm	AER violation[b]
Advisory actions (warning letters)			
2/25/11	6/17/11	BioSan	Did not include domestic contact information to report an adverse event on product label and did not submit mandatory AER to FDA within 15 days.
7/13/11	10/11/11	Nordimex	Did not include contact information to report an adverse event on product label.
12/7/2011	4/2/12	Theta Brothers Sports Nutrition	
Regulatory actions (injunction)			
4/22/11	3/9/12	ATF Fitness Products and Manufacturing ATF Dedicated Excellence, Inc.	Did not report serious AERs to FDA.
Regulatory actions (import refusals)[c]			
6/27/11	9/7/11	Bio-minerals	Did not include domestic contact information to report an adverse event on product label.
6/22/11	9/15/11	Hayashi Industria E Comercio D	
5/31/11	9/20/11	Forza Vitale Italia SRL	
5/9/11	10/4/11	Guangzhou Tian Yi Import & Export Company Limited	
10/9/11	12/5/11	Metabolics Limited: FDA refused 7 different imported product shipments from this firm on this date.	
4/20/11	12/12/11	Tatsuhiko Kono	
4/19/11	12/12/11	Hipernatural.Com	
1/31/11	8/12/11	Hersol Manufacturing Laboratories	
12/29/09	6/16/10	Stephen Health Agency	

Source: GAO analysis of FDA data.

[a] For warning letters and injunctions, the initiation date is the date the shipment was offered for entry into U.S. commerce. For import refusals, the initiation date is the date that the import shipment was processed by the U.S. Customs Service.

[b] Data provided to GAO as of April 13, 2012.

[c] The refusals shown in this table are those for which FDA specifically cited an AER-related violation, not other more general types of violations, such as labeling.

According to FDA officials, inspections are the primary way FDA identifies and develops direct evidence of noncompliance with AER requirements. However, FDA and others have identified noncompliant firms through other surveillance actions. Specifically, FDA can also identify and act on noncompliance with some AER requirements through Internet monitoring. For example, in March 2012, after reviewing a product label on a firm's website, FDA sent a warning letter to the firm for failing to include domestic contact information to report an adverse event on the product label. In addition, in October 2012, the HHS Inspector General reported that 20 percent of a judgmental sample of 127 dietary supplement products purchased from retail stores or online lacked contact information to report adverse events.[50] This study is not representative of the dietary supplement industry, but it indicates that compliance with AER requirements remains an issue for some firms. According to Inspector General officials, the Inspector General provided a list of the noncompliant firms to FDA for the agency's review.[51]

FDA can estimate noncompliance to some extent using its known advisory and regulatory actions specific to AER requirements, but the actual number of noncompliant firms may not be fully reflected by these data. For example, an FDA official said that companies that deliberately adulterate supplement products with active pharmaceutical ingredients to increase their potency probably are also noncompliant with AER requirements, but FDA can only act on those violations for which it has direct evidence. Specifically, FDA may be able to identify a supplement adulterated with such ingredients from voluntary AERs submitted by consumers, health care practitioners, or others, but it would need to perform an inspection to determine noncompliance with most AER requirements.[52] FDA may also have difficulty targeting such firms for inspections because they may not register with FDA as required by law. For example, in its October 2012 report, the HHS Inspector General found that 28 percent, or 22 of the 79 companies in its sample, had not registered with FDA as required.[53] FDA officials believe that the rate of noncompliance is greater than the regulatory action data indicate, but these officials told us that they have not estimated what the noncompliance rate might be because they cannot make assumptions about the behavior of firms.

FDA Has Used AERs for Some Actions but May Have Opportunities to Expand its Use of AERs

FDA has used AERs for some consumer protection actions (i.e., surveillance, advisory, and regulatory actions), although the exact number is largely unknown. FDA officials said that most AERs do not initiate or support consumer protection actions because it is difficult to establish causality based on the limited information in an AER. However, FDA does not collect information on how it uses AERs for its consumer protection actions; FDA could draw on such information to assess whether AERs are being used to their fullest extent for consumer protection. FDA could also expand electronic reporting to firms for mandatory AERs, which could reduce data entry costs and make more program funds available for analysis. FDA is not required to provide information to the public about potential safety concerns from dietary supplement AERs as it is for drugs. Making such information public, if consistent with disclosure provisions in existing law, could expand FDA's use of AERs and improve consumer awareness and understanding of potential health problems associated with supplements.

FDA Has Used AERs to Initiate or Support Some Consumer Protection Actions

FDA has used AERs to initiate or support some consumer protection actions, but the exact number of reports used and actions taken is largely unknown. According to FDA officials, FDA uses AERs to initiate or support certain consumer protection actions on a case-by-case basis, such as inspections, consumer alerts, and recalls. FDA officials said they also use AERs to provide data for general research on products and ingredients. However, it is difficult to identify the full extent to which FDA uses AERs to initiate or support consumer protection actions because FDA does not have mechanisms in place to systematically monitor the relationship between AERs and these actions.

According to FDA officials, most AERs that are received by FDA do not initiate or support consumer protection actions because it is difficult to establish a causal link between supplements and reported health problems based on the limited information available within an individual AER.[54] Specifically, AERs typically do not include details on the consumer's medical history or other products, such as prescription drugs that the consumer may have consumed simultaneously. Details such as underlying medical conditions and allergies are requested as part of the reporting process, but FDA officials said that there is generally a lot of missing information in both voluntary and mandatory AERs.[55] For example, age was not available in 32 percent of the dietary supplement AERs that FDA received, and pregnancy status was not available in 98 percent of the AERs involving females. Additionally, because AERs represent a reported association in time between a supplement and a health problem, FDA must first establish the likelihood that the supplement caused the health problem before considering it in the context of consumer protection actions. However, FDA officials told us that AERs may contain inconclusive and often inconsistent data from which it may be impossible to draw consistently strong inferences. For example, FDA was only able to establish a "certain" relationship between the supplement and reported health problem in 3 percent (212 of 6,307) of the AERs. For 67 percent (4,211 of 6,307) of the AERs, FDA could not determine whether the supplement caused the reported health problem because the AER contained insufficient information.[56] Additionally, FDA officials told us that AERs may be complete but contain little evidence necessary for FDA to take action. For example, FDA needs to demonstrate a known effect from the timing and dosage of the supplement product in question.

Because FDA has the burden of proof to demonstrate that a product carries a significant or unreasonable risk of injury or illness for dietary supplement products on the market prior to 1994 under current law, the limited information available to FDA based on an individual AER does not usually provide enough evidence to take action. FDA officials said it is more common to identify potential problems after analyzing a cluster of AERs, along with evidence from other sources, such as published research. For example, a subject matter expert in the Division of Dietary Supplement Programs may track a cluster of AERs separately in a spreadsheet and then forward the information to CFSAN's Office of Compliance if the expert believes that a regulatory compliance issue or potential health issue may be present.[57] The Office of Compliance, in turn, may initiate an advisory or regulatory action, or coordinate with FDA's Office of Regulatory Affairs to conduct additional surveillance, such as an inspection prior to taking an advisory or regulatory action. However, accumulating enough evidence to discern a clear relationship between a specific product or ingredient and a reported health problem may take receiving a number of AERs over a span of months or years. For example, because liver-related problems associated with Hydroxycut™ were reported infrequently, it took 7 years for FDA to establish a clear relationship between the Hydroxycut™ products and liver disease.[58] After establishing a causal relationship in 2009, FDA discussed a voluntary recall with the manufacturer of Hydroxycut™ products and issued a consumer advisory against using these products.

To estimate the extent to which FDA uses AERs to initiate or support consumer protection actions, we compared firm and product names identified in both mandatory AERs and FDA actions to determine if an AER preceded a consumer protection action related to a dietary supplement. Out of the roughly 4,700 consumer protection actions related to dietary supplements that we reviewed, we found 61 actions (about 1 percent) where FDA received a mandatory AER for the same firm or product prior to taking action, as detailed in table 4, which supports FDA officials' assessment that most AERs do not support consumer protection actions.[59] However, we could not verify that all of the 61 actions we identified were necessarily initiated or supported by AERs because FDA does not systematically monitor this information, and officials could not verify a relationship between the AERs and the actions taken prior to the issuance of this report.[60] Additionally, our analysis does not include situations where FDA used AERs to inform its decisions but did not take formal action.

Table 4. Mandatory AERs Preceding Certain FDA Consumer Protection Actions Related to Dietary Supplements, 2008 through 2011

Type of action	Description
Surveillance	We identified 47 inspections for firms also listed in an AER, representing 6 percent of all dietary supplement inspections from 2008 through 2011. These inspections included compliance, surveillance, and follow-up inspections.
Advisory	We identified 3 advisory actions for firms or products also listed in an AER, representing less than 1 percent of dietary supplement advisory actions from 2008 through 2011. The advisory actions included two warning letters and 1 consumer alert for firms or products also listed in an AER.
Regulatory	We identified 11 regulatory actions for firms or products also listed in an AER, representing less than 1 percent of dietary supplement regulatory actions from 2008 through 2011. The regulatory actions included 8 import refusals and 3 voluntary product recalls initiated by firms.

Source: GAO analysis of FDA data.

Note: We also reviewed seizures, injunctions, criminal investigations, and industry alerts to identify consumer protection actions that might have been preceded by a mandatory AER. However, we did not find any matches between mandatory AERs and these actions.

According to our analysis, we identified 47 inspections for firms also listed in an AER, representing 6 percent of all dietary supplement inspections from 2008 and 2011. Similarly, we found 3 advisory actions for firms also listed in an AER, which represent less than 1 percent of all such actions. Two of the advisory actions were warning letters for noncompliance with CGMP requirements, and another was a consumer alert on Hydroxycut™ products. We also identified 11 regulatory actions for firms also listed in an AER, representing less than 1 percent of all such actions. The regulatory actions included 8 import refusals and 3 product recalls, most of which were for Hydroxycut™ products. (See app. II for more information on consumer protection actions.) FDA officials told us they also use AERs to monitor the results of these actions. For example, if FDA issued a warning letter to a firm based on violations of CGMP requirements during an inspection, receipt of subsequent AERs may indicate that the firm has not rectified its practices. Similarly, if FDA receives an AER for a product that FDA has removed from the market by a regulatory action such as a recall, FDA's receipt of AERs subsequent to the initial action indicates to FDA that further action may be needed.

More Information on How FDA Uses AERs May Help FDA Expand Their Use

FDA has limited information on how it uses AERs to initiate and support its consumer protection actions; such information could improve FDA's ability to assess whether the agency is using AERs to their fullest extent in this capacity and make improvements as needed. For example, prior work has shown that agencies can use data on performance to identify and mitigate problems, allocate resources, and improve effectiveness.[61] Currently, FDA uses six separate data management systems to monitor the consumer protection actions we reviewed apart from AERs, as outlined in table 5.

FDA can track each type of action in its respective data management system and tracks certain identifying information, such as firm name, across all the systems. However, FDA generally does not track AERs across these systems. Specifically, within the six data management systems we reviewed, we found that FDA only tracks the relationship between consumer complaints and AERs. Without having a mechanism to follow an AER through to other actions, FDA misses the opportunity to assess how frequently AERs initiate or support consumer protection actions and to identify ways to potentially broaden their use. For example, FDA internal guidance states that AERs can be used to demonstrate potential health risks associated with violative conditions found during other surveillance activities, such as inspections, and be part of the evidence gathered to support regulatory actions. Establishing the potential for harm is particularly important for dietary supplements because the burden of proof to demonstrate a significant or unreasonable risk of illness or injury prior to removing a product from the market through a regulatory action falls upon FDA. However, by not tracking the relationship between AERs and its other data management systems, FDA cannot systematically identify the extent to which AERS were used in this capacity. Having such information could improve FDA's and policymakers' abilities to make fully informed decisions about resource allocation and AERs' future role in FDA's consumer protection activities related to dietary supplements.

Furthermore, unlike other FDA-regulated products, dietary supplement firms cannot submit mandatory AERs electronically. Rather, they must submit these AERs in hard copy by mail. FDA's requirement that firms submit mandatory AERs in hard copy form by mail—which must be entered manually into the CAERS database by CAERS staff—may reduce the AER system's effectiveness by diverting resources to data entry rather than analysis. According to CFSAN officials, FDA has plans to expand electronic reporting to mandatory AERs for dietary supplements in mid-2014 as part of its Safety Reporting Portal Program. However, FDA had similar plans at the time of our prior report in 2009 that have not been realized yet.

Providing Information to the Public on Dietary Supplement AERs May Improve Consumer Understanding

Communicating effectively about risks related to dietary supplements is a key part of FDA's mission to protect and promote public health, according to FDA's strategic plan. Specifically, helping consumers better understand the risks and benefits of regulated products is a key part of FDA's responsibilities, as described in the agency's 2009 *Strategic Plan for Risk Communication*. This plan outlines a number of strategies to improve communication, including identifying and filling gaps in key areas of risk communication and improving the effectiveness of FDA's website and web tools. In addition, guidance from the Office of Management and Budget and HHS, as well as our prior work, has emphasized providing greater transparency and participation of federal agencies in publishing government information online.[62] However, unlike drugs and certain biologic products—where FDA is required to provide information about identified potential safety concerns by law—little information on potential safety concerns from dietary supplement AERs is publicly available and accessible to consumers, health care practitioners, and others.[63] Specifically, for dietary supplement AERs, FDA generally provides information on its website on the number of mandatory AERs it received and the number of unique firm names from all mandatory AERs on a monthly basis. This aggregated information, which is located under FDA's performance measures for CFSAN and is not directly linked with the dietary supplement web pages, does not provide any indication to consumers of potential risks associated with specific dietary supplements.[64] In November 2012, FDA also posted information on its website about individual AERs the agency had received from January 2004 through October 2012 associated with four types of "energy drinks"—three of which were sold as dietary supplements, one as a conventional food. Individuals may also request information about adverse events related to dietary supplements by submitting a Freedom of Information Act request to FDA.

Table 5. Examples of FDA Data Management Systems to Monitor Consumer Protection Actions Related to Dietary Supplements

Data management system	Action monitored[a]	FDA office
Automated Investigative Management System	Criminal investigations	Office of Regulatory Affairs
CFSAN Adverse Event Reporting System (CAERS)	AERs	CFSAN
Compliance Management System	Warning letters, seizures, and injunctions	Office of Regulatory Affairs
Field Accomplishments and Compliance Tracking System	Consumer complaints and inspections	Office of Crisis Management and Office of Regulatory Affairs
Operational and Administrative System for Import Support	Import screenings and refusals	Office of Regulatory Affairs
Recall Enterprise System	Product recalls	Office of Regulatory Affairs

Source: GAO analysis of FDA documents.

[a] This column includes those consumer protection actions that we reviewed as part of this report and not necessarily all of the activities monitored by the data management systems.

According to FDA officials, there are certain disclosure provisions within the Federal Food, Drug, and Cosmetic Act that limit FDA's ability to provide unredacted information on AERs related to dietary supplements.[65] However, FDA provides detailed aggregated analysis, including a list of products with potential safety concerns, and raw disaggregated data on AERs related to drugs and certain biologic products on its website, even though some of the same and similar disclosure provisions may apply to such products. Specifically, in the disaggregated data on prescription drugs, FDA redacts names and other information that would identify the individual reporting the adverse event and, occasionally, information on any ongoing clinical studies or other pending actions, if applicable. The publicly available disaggregated data, including product names and health problems, are then used for health and medical research. For example, researchers have used data available from prescription drug AERs to study cardiovascular risk,[66] bladder cancer,[67] and tachycardia (accelerated heart rate).[68] FDA officials told us that they use dietary supplement-related AERs to conduct safety-related research on dietary supplement ingredients, and other government researchers have used AERs in a similar capacity. According to agency officials, FDA already applies a redaction approach to prescription drug AERs that meets the nondisclosure provisions within the Federal Food, Drug, and Cosmetic Act that apply to dietary supplement AERs. An FDA official has stated publicly that the agency is exploring ways to expand the amount of publicly available information about AERs for dietary supplements.[69] To the extent that FDA can do so under existing law—providing greater information about dietary supplement AERs to the public, such as potential safety concerns and redacted data on its website—could create opportunities for external researchers to use AERs and to improve consumer awareness and understanding of potential health problems associated with dietary supplements.

FDA Has Partially Implemented All of Our 2009 Recommendations

FDA has partially implemented each of our four recommendations from our 2009 report on dietary supplements.[70] Table 6 summarizes our 2009 recommendations and FDA or congressional action.

Table 6. 2009 GAO Recommendations on Dietary Supplements and FDA or Congressional Action

GAO recommendation	FDA or congressional action
FDA should request additional authority to: (1) require firms to self-identify as dietary supplement firms as part of existing registration requirements, provide information on the products they sell, and update this information annually and (2) require firms to report all adverse events.	(1) FDA officials told us they requested additional authority as part of the FDA Food Safety and Modernization Act of 2011 (FSMA) to modify the list of required food categories that FDA uses to identify firms by industry as part of existing registration requirements. In August 2012, FDA published draft guidance expanding the list of food categories required at registration to include dietary supplement categories that were previously optional. FDA issued final guidance in October 2012. Requiring dietary supplement firms to provide information on the products they sell has been part of multiple proposed legislative efforts but has not become law.[a] (2) Mandatory reporting of all adverse events for dietary supplement firms was proposed in S. 3002, the Dietary Supplement Safety Act of 2010, sponsored by Senators McCain and Dorgan, but did not pass the Senate.
FDA should issue new dietary ingredient (NDI) notification guidance.	As part of FSMA, FDA was required to issue draft NDI notification guidance no later than 180 days after enactment. FDA published its draft guidance in July 2011. An FDA official said the agency is still reviewing the more than 7,000 comments it received in response to the draft guidance.
FDA should issue guidance to industry clarifying when products should be marketed as dietary supplements or conventional foods formulated with added dietary ingredients.	FDA issued draft guidance to industry clarifying when liquid products may be marketed as dietary supplements or conventional foods with novel ingredients in December 2009.[b] FDA has indicated it is developing final guidance but has not set a time frame for its issuance.
FDA should coordinate with stakeholder groups involved in consumer outreach to identify, implement, and assess the effectiveness of additional mechanisms for educating consumers about dietary supplements.	FDA coordinated with stakeholder groups by expanding its partnership with the website WebMD™ to include vitamin- and supplement-specific pages and formed new stakeholder partnerships with EverydayHealth™ and Drugs.com™ websites to educate consumers about dietary supplements. FDA also expanded the consumer education content on its own website and implemented new mechanisms for reaching consumers, such as a Really Simple Syndication (RSS) feed on tainted (i.e., adulterated) products marketed as dietary supplements and consumer updates. FDA collects information about the number of RSS feed subscribers and page views that can be used to measure distribution.[c]

Source: GAO.

[a] The Food Safety Enhancement Act of 2009, H.R. 2749, 111th Cong. (passed by the House of Representatives July 30, 2009); the Dietary Supplement Safety Act of 2010, S.3002, 111th Cong. (sponsored by Senators McCain and Dorgan); the Dietary Supplement Labeling Act of 2011, S. 1310, 112th Cong.(sponsored by Senators Durbin and Blumenthal). In addition to these efforts, individual

legislators have also introduced amendments with provisions regarding product registration to other legislation under consideration.

[b] The Federal Food, Drug, and Cosmetic Act (21 U.S.C. §§ 321(s), 348(a) generally requires that when a company adds an ingredient to a food product, that ingredient must either be generally recognized as safe (GRAS) or go through FDA's review and approval process as a food additive. The GRAS standard is defined as a general recognition among qualified experts that the substance is reasonably certain to be safe under conditions of its intended use. See GAO, *FDA Should Strengthen Its Oversight of Food Ingredients Determined to Be Generally Recognized as Safe (GRAS),* GAO-10-246 (Washington, D.C.: Feb. 3, 2010) for more information.

[c] According to FDA data, as of July 31, 2012, the number of page views for the dietary supplement pages ranged from 22,687 views for the "Tainted Sexual Enhancement Products" page to 249,783 views for the "Overview of Dietary Supplements" page. There are 58,633 subscribers to the tainted products marketed as dietary supplements govdelivery e-mail subscription service. There are 135 subscribers to the tainted products RSS feed and 828 subscribers to the consumer update RSS feed. According to FDA officials, FDA is precluded from collecting similar metrics for content on its partnership pages owing to Freedom of Information Act restrictions on the release of commercial confidential information.

FDA officials said that the agency is planning to issue final guidance and complete implementation for most of our recommendations, but they do not have a time frame for completion. Specifically, FDA officials said they plan to issue final NDI guidance, but they are still reviewing more than 7,000 distinct comments they received in response to the draft NDI guidance issued in July 2011. Furthermore, although FDA officials have indicated they intend to issue final guidance clarifying whether a liquid product may be labeled and marketed as a dietary supplement and possibly issuing similar guidance for non-liquid products, they have not indicated to us where they are in this process. Regarding our recommendation on consumer outreach, FDA officials said that assessing the effectiveness of its outreach efforts through the WebMD™ and other partnerships, consumer updates, and fact sheets on dietary supplement safety issues would require extensive consumer research, which would have to be considered in light of FDA's limited resources and competing priorities.

Consequently, regulatory uncertainty remains an issue for areas covered only by draft guidance. As we have previously reported, without final NDI guidance in place, firms may not notify FDA before marketing products with ingredients that have drastically different safety profiles than their historical use.[71] In addition, "energy drinks"—some of which are marketed as beverages and others as dietary supplements—have raised concerns about potential health risks among consumer advocacy groups, academics, government agencies, and members of Congress.[72] Specifically, concerns raised by these groups include the potential health risks associated with the level of caffeine in these products, the combination of caffeine and botanical ingredients with stimulant properties in these products, and their popularity with youth. Two of the four top-selling brands of energy drinks in 2012, as identified by a market research firm, were marketed as dietary supplements, while the others were marketed as beverages. As we noted in our 2009 report, this boundary matters because the safety standard for a certain ingredient in food is different than that for the same ingredient when it is used as a dietary ingredient in a dietary supplement. The differences in how products are regulated may lead to circumstances when an ingredient would not be allowed to be added to a product if it was labeled as a conventional food but would be allowed in the identical product if it was labeled as a dietary supplement. Even without final guidance to industry, the agency has issued warning letters to firms for violations related to NDI notifications and the distinction between liquid dietary supplements and conventional foods on a case-by-case basis. With clear guidance to industry about these issues, firms may have the information necessary to guide appropriate product development—including the development of safety information—and marketing, and FDA's enforcement burden in these areas may be reduced as a result. Moreover, by assessing its outreach efforts, FDA would have information on whether its new approaches are effective, which could help FDA target future efforts, particularly in the area of increasing voluntary adverse event reporting.

CONCLUSION

Because of an increase in mandatory AERs, the number of AERs FDA has received since 2008 for dietary supplements has more than doubled, and FDA has used AERs to initiate and support some consumer protection actions. However, consumers and others may not be voluntarily reporting information to FDA on all adverse events that occur, although they may be contacting poison centers about some of these events. FDA officials said that their greatest challenge to identifying potential safety concerns from AERs is the relatively small number of AERs the agency receives, and that—depending on its review of the poison center data—FDA may benefit from obtaining access to these data for analysis. According to FDA officials, negotiations to access the data are ongoing at the HHS level but, as of December 2012, the results of these negotiations were still pending.

Furthermore, although FDA has used AERs for some consumer protection actions, FDA may have opportunities to expand its use of AERs. FDA does not systematically collect information on how it uses AERs; such information could improve FDA's ability to assess whether the agency is using AERs to their fullest extent in consumer protection actions and make improvements as needed. For example, FDA guidance states that AERs can be used to demonstrate potential health risks associated with violations found during other surveillance activities, such as inspections, and be part of the evidence gathered to support regulatory actions. However, by not tracking the relationship between AERs and its other data management systems, FDA cannot identify the extent to which AERS were used in this capacity. Having such information may also improve FDA's and policymakers' abilities to make fully informed decisions about resource allocation and AERs' future role in FDA's consumer protection activities related to dietary supplements.

In addition, FDA's process for collecting and managing mandatory AERs could be more efficient because dietary supplement firms, unlike other FDA-regulated products, cannot submit mandatory AERs electronically. Rather, they must submit these AERs in hard copy by mail. FDA officials said that they have plans to expand electronic reporting; however, FDA had similar plans in place at the time we issued our 2009 report that were never realized. To the extent that FDA can do so under existing law, providing greater information about dietary supplement AERs to the public—such as identified potential safety concerns and redacted data on its website—could create opportunities for external researchers to use AERs and to improve consumer awareness and understanding of potential health problems associated with dietary supplements.

Moreover, regulatory uncertainty remains an issue in two key areas of dietary supplement regulation because FDA has not set a time frame for issuing final guidance for draft NDI notification guidance and draft guidance clarifying when liquid products may be marketed as dietary supplements or conventional foods with added ingredients or for issuing similar guidance for nonliquid products. With final guidance in these areas, firms may be able to make more informed marketing and product development decisions, including the development of safety information, and ultimately FDA's enforcement burden in these areas may be reduced as a result.

RECOMMENDATIONS FOR EXECUTIVE ACTION

To enhance FDA's ability to use AERs and to oversee dietary supplement products, we recommend that the Secretary of the Department of Health and Human Services direct the Commissioner of FDA to take the following five actions:

- Continue efforts to explore all possible options to obtain poison center data if the agency determines that the data could inform FDA's ability to identify potential safety concerns from adverse event reports for dietary supplements.
- Incorporate a mechanism to collect information on when AERs are used to support and inform consumer protection actions (i.e., surveillance, advisory, and regulatory actions).
- Implement the agency's efforts to facilitate industry reporting of mandatory AERs electronically.
- Determine what additional information FDA can provide to the public about dietary supplement AERs consistent with existing law and make the information publicly available and readily accessible on its website.
- Establish a time frame for issuing final guidance for the draft (1) NDI guidance and (2) guidance clarifying whether a liquid product may be labeled and marketed as a dietary supplement or as a conventional food with added ingredients.

AGENCY COMMENTS

We provided the Secretary of Health and Human Services with a draft of this report for review and comment. We received a written response from the Assistant Secretary for Legislation that included comments from FDA. FDA generally agreed with each of the report's recommendations. HHS also sent us technical comments on behalf of FDA, which we incorporated as appropriate.

J. Alfredo Gómez
Director, Natural Resources and Environment

APPENDIX I: OBJECTIVES, SCOPE, AND METHODOLOGY

Our objectives were to determine the (1) number of adverse event reports (AER) the Food and Drug Administration (FDA) has received since 2008, the source of these reports, and the types of products identified; (2) actions FDA has taken to ensure that firms are complying with new reporting requirements; (3) extent to which FDA is using AERs for its consumer protection actions; and (4) extent to which FDA has implemented GAO's 2009 recommendations for enhancing FDA oversight of dietary supplements.

For this report, dietary supplement refers to a product intended for consumption as defined in the Dietary Supplement Health and Education Act of 1994 (DSHEA)—products that, among other things, are intended for ingestion to supplement the diet, labeled as a dietary supplement and not represented as a conventional food or as a sole item of a meal or diet. They must also contain one or more dietary ingredients. This definition covers supplements for human consumption. We did not examine FDA's oversight of products that would otherwise meet the definition of a dietary supplement in DSHEA but are intended for veterinary use. We also did not examine FDA's oversight of products that would otherwise meet the definition of a dietary supplement in DSHEA but are available only by prescription. We did include products that are marketed as dietary supplements but that have been deliberately adulterated (e.g., tainted with active ingredients in FDA-approved drugs or their analogues to increase their potency). Although such products may not meet the legal definition of a dietary supplement because they contain prescription drug ingredients, we included them in our review because these products are often marketed as dietary supplements and can cause serious health problems.

To determine the number of AERs that FDA received, the source of the reports, and the types of products identified, we obtained and analyzed FDA data on the number and type of AERs received since the reporting requirements went into effect in January 2008 through December 2011. Some of the data and analyses were provided by FDA in aggregate form, although FDA also provided us with disaggregate data on serious AERs. We supplemented our initial analysis with updated data on the number of AERs that FDA received between January 1 and September 30, 2012. To count the number of AERs associated with a unique firm or product, we sorted the data by firm name then manually reviewed the names to identify firms with similar or related names. We used the same approach for products, reasoning that products with similar formulations and active ingredients should be grouped together because they would cause similar reactions in consumers and may be manufactured in the same facility.[73] In some cases, we performed additional Internet research to verify the accuracy of a match between a firm or product name. We also reviewed and analyzed data on calls about adverse events related to dietary supplements to poison centers from annual reports of the American Association of Poison Control Centers (AAPCC) from 2008 through 2010. Because poison centers classify certain dietary supplement products differently than FDA, such as including homeopathic agents as dietary supplements, we worked with AAPCC and FDA officials to make the appropriate adjustments to the data to make them comparable to FDA AERs. Similarly, because FDA officials told us that AERs are primarily associated with product use as directed, we adjusted the poison center data to include only those cases where an individual experienced an adverse reaction when using the product as directed and excluded reports resulting from misuse, abuse, or accidental ingestion. To assess the reliability of these data, we reviewed related documentation, reviewed internal controls, and worked with agency or AAPCC officials to identify any data problems. For the FDA data on serious AERs, which we received in disaggregate form, we examined the data to identify obvious errors or inconsistencies. We also reviewed FDA's laws, rules, and regulations relevant to collecting and maintaining AERs. We determined the data to be sufficiently reliable for the purposes of this report.

To determine actions FDA has taken to ensure that firms are complying with new reporting requirements, we reviewed FDA's procedures, planning documents, and guidance and obtained and analyzed data on FDA's oversight activities, such as inspections, advisory, and regulatory actions, to identify which of these actions were related to monitoring or enforcing firms' compliance. Specifically, we obtained aggregate data on the number of dietary supplement inspections from January 1, 2008, through September 30, 2012 and analyzed record-level data on the type and results of dietary supplement inspections FDA conducted from 2008 through 2011 from FDA's Field Accomplishments and Compliance Tracking System. To determine the number of AER violations observed during inspections, we obtained and analyzed aggregate data from FDA's Turbo EIR system on inspection observations from fiscal year 2008 through fiscal year 2012. To determine the number of advisory and regulatory actions related to AER violations from January 1, 2008 through December 31, 2011, we obtained and analyzed data and documents on warning letters, seizures, and injunctions from FDA's Compliance Management System and FDA's online warning letter database; Class I recalls[74] from FDA's Recall Enterprise System and other safety-related recalls identified from press releases on FDA's Recalls - Health Fraud web page and Recalls, Market Withdrawals, and Safety Alerts web page[75]; import refusals from FDA's Operational and Administrative System for Import Support; and prosecutions with charges filed, convictions, or settlements reached in FDA's Automated Investigative Management System. We also reviewed individual firm inspection reports for examples of specific observations found during dietary supplement inspections, and accompanied FDA investigators on an inspection of a dietary supplement manufacturing facility. To assess the reliability of data supporting this objective, we reviewed related documentation, internal controls, examined the data to identify obvious errors or inconsistencies, traced data back to source documents, and identified and removed data that were outside the scope of our review, such as data related to products for animal or prescription uses, or data that did not meet the definition of dietary supplement used for this report, as described above. We determined the data to be sufficiently reliable for the purposes of this report.

To determine the extent to which FDA is using AERs to initiate and support its consumer protection actions, we matched firm and product names from mandatory AERs against firm and product names in the following FDA consumer protection actions from January 2008 through December 2011: inspections, consumer alerts, industry advisories, warning letters, seizures and injunctions, import refusals, safety-related recalls, and prosecutions.[76] The matching process was necessary because FDA does not track how it uses AERs to initiate or support consumer protection actions across its other data systems. Because CFSAN officials told us that product and firm names are not standardized within the CFSAN Adverse Event Reporting System (CAERS) or across FDA's systems, we used statistical software to build wild-card searches to identify potential matches and then reviewed each potential match to confirm or reject potential matches.

Specifically, we used an analytical software function that measures spelling differences between words to determine the likelihood that firm and product names from two data sets matched and to generate possible matches between AERs and actions. The statistical software returns a numeric value indicating how closely related the names are. After reviewing the initial results, we established a threshold for matching that gave us confidence we were capturing most of the potential matches and excluding those that were definitely not a match.

The matches were then manually reviewed to confirm or reject potential matches. For matched records, we determined whether an AER was received prior to the consumer protection action, as an indicator that the AER may have contributed to FDA's decision to take action. For matched records, we tabulated both the number of AERs that contributed to each action, and the number of actions that matched AERs. We verified the appropriateness of this approach with FDA officials prior to conducting the analysis and provided a list of matches to FDA for their verification. We also reviewed FDA's guidance and procedures relevant to using AERs to initiate or support surveillance, advisory, and regulatory actions.

To determine the extent to which FDA has implemented GAO's 2009 recommendations for enhancing FDA oversight of dietary supplements, we reviewed FDA's laws, planning documents, and guidance. We reviewed proposed legislation to expand FDA's oversight authority for dietary supplements. We also obtained data on the extent to which FDA's web-based consumer outreach initiatives were distributed.

In addition, to address all of our objectives, we reviewed relevant studies related to dietary supplements, adverse event reporting, industry compliance, and using poison center data for public health surveillance, among others. We reviewed the methodology for each of these studies and assessed them for reasonableness in accordance with our objectives.

We also interviewed officials from several FDA offices, including FDA's Center for Food Safety and Applied Nutrition (CFSAN) who receive and analyze AERs, officials from FDA's Division of Dietary Supplements Program, officials from the Office of Regulatory Affairs familiar with FDA's field operations and regulatory actions related to dietary supplements, and officials from the Center for Drug Evaluation and Research. We interviewed a wide range of stakeholders, including officials from federal agencies, industry and trade organizations, and consumer advocacy groups. At the federal level outside of FDA, we met with officials from the Department of Health and Human Services' (HHS) Centers for Disease Control and Prevention, the National Institutes of Health, and the Federal Trade Commission. At the industry level, we spoke with representatives from the American Herbal Products Association, the Council for Responsible Nutrition, and the Natural Products Association.

At the consumer advocacy level, we met with representatives from the Center for Science in the Public Interest, Consumers Union, and Public Citizen. We also spoke with representatives from the American Association of Poison Control Centers.

We conducted this performance audit from December 2011 to March 2013 in accordance with generally accepted government auditing standards. Those standards require that we plan and perform the audit to obtain sufficient, appropriate evidence to provide a reasonable basis for our findings and conclusions based on our audit objectives. We believe that the evidence obtained provides a reasonable basis for our findings and conclusions based on our audit objectives.

APPENDIX II: DATA ON FDA'S CONSUMER PROTECTION ACTIONS RELATED TO DIETARY SUPPLEMENTS

This appendix combines data collected during this review with data from our prior report to provide additional detail on FDA's actions to identify and respond to safety concerns related to dietary supplements.[77]

Data on FDA's Surveillance Actions Related to Dietary Supplements

FDA actions to identify safety concerns related to dietary supplements include receiving and analyzing adverse event reports and consumer complaints and conducting inspections.

Data on Adverse Event Reports Related to Dietary Supplements

Incorporating data from our prior report, figure 7 shows the number of dietary supplement-related AERs entered into FDA's database from January 1, 2003, through September 30, 2012. As shown in 2008, mandatory reporting had an immediate impact on the number of dietary supplement-related AERs FDA received.

Data on Consumer Complaints Related to Dietary Supplements

Incorporating data from our prior report, figure 8 shows the number of dietary supplement-related consumer complaints with adverse event results or reported symptoms FDA received from January 1, 2002, through December 31, 2011. Consumer complaints are not limited to adverse events. For example, consumers may report a complaint if one or more pills in a product are discolored.

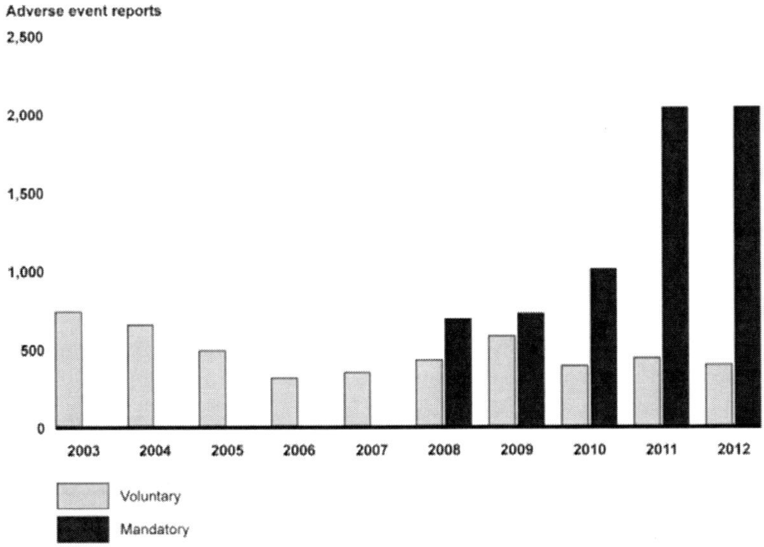

Source: GAO analysis of FDA data.

Note: Although mandatory reporting went into effect on December 22, 2007, FDA did not receive its first mandatory report until January 2008. In some cases, FDA received both voluntary and mandatory AERs for the same adverse event. To avoid double-counting, we included these cases in the mandatory AER total. FDA received from 12 to 24 AERs per year as both mandatory and voluntary from January 1, 2008, through September 30, 2012.

Figure 7. Voluntary and Mandatory AERs Related to Dietary Supplements Received by FDA, 2003 through September 30, 2012.

Data on Inspections Related to Dietary Supplements

Incorporating data from our prior report, figure 9 shows the number of dietary supplement inspections conducted by FDA or its state partners and the proportion of these inspections where the investigator identified problems from January 1, 2002, through December 31, 2011. For our determination for whether FDA identified a problem during an inspection, we included all inspections where the district determined that: (1) official action is indicated, (2) voluntary action is indicated, and (3) the case should be referred to CFSAN's Office of Compliance. We also included all cases where the investigator completed an inspectional observation form—a form used by FDA to document concerns observed during inspections. The items listed on these forms are preliminary and vary in severity. Each inspection was counted only once.

Figure 10 shows the type of dietary supplement inspections conducted from January 1, 2008, through December 31, 2011. Complaint inspections are conducted to investigate consumer complaints about a firm. Follow-up inspections are conducted to assess a firm's progress after an advisory or regulatory action such as a warning letter or recall. Compliance inspections are "for-cause" inspections to investigate specific compliance issues. Surveillance inspections are routine inspections that generally assess whether a firm is following dietary supplement good manufacturing practices, as applicable. An inspection may include product examinations, sampling and testing, as well as the inspection of the firm and facility involved with dietary supplements, according to FDA officials.

Data on FDA's Advisory and Regulatory Actions Related to Dietary Supplements

FDA actions to respond to safety concerns related to dietary supplements include issuing warning letters to dietary supplement firms, working with firms on recalls, and refusing imports.

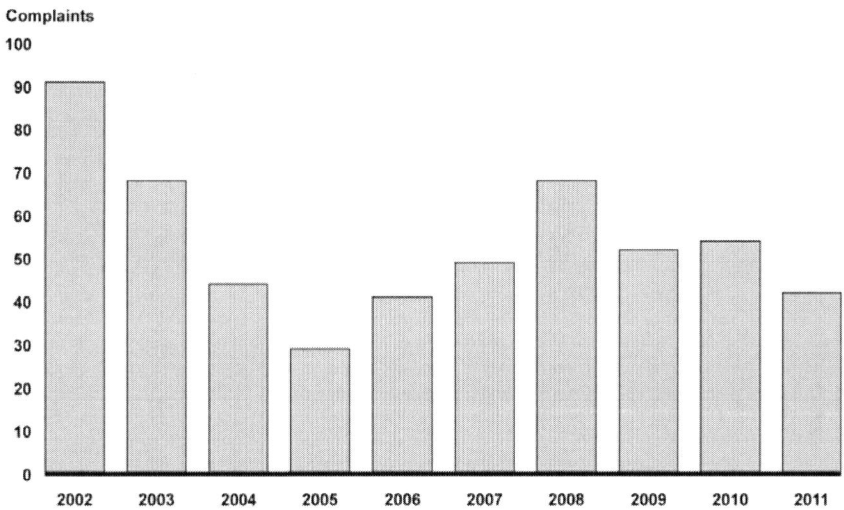

Source: GAO analysis of FDA data.

Figure 8. Dietary Supplement-Related Consumer Complaints with Adverse Event Results or Reported Symptoms Received by FDA, 2002 through 2011.

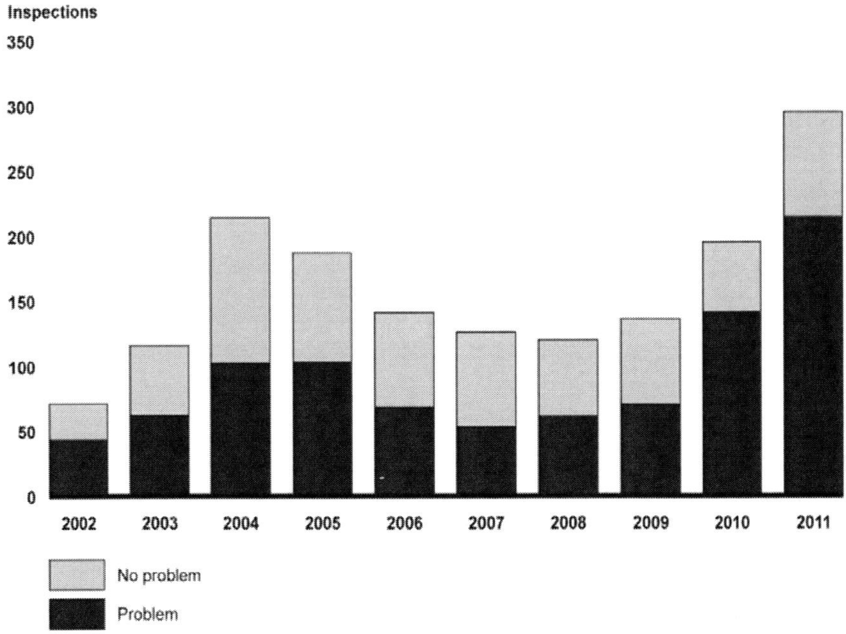

Source: GAO analysis of FDA data.

Note: Current good manufacturing practices (CGMP) specific to dietary supplement firms were phased in by firm size from 2008 to 2010. For firms with 500 or more full-time equivalent employees, they became effective in June 2008; for firms with at least 20 but fewer than 500 full-time equivalent employees, they became effective in June 2009; and for firms with fewer than 20 full-time equivalent employees they became effective in June 2010. According to FDA officials, prior to the establishment of dietary supplement-specific CGMPs, FDA inspected dietary supplement firms according to food CGMPs.

Figure 9. Proportion of Dietary Supplement Inspections for Which FDA Identified Problems or Concerns, 2002 through 2011.

Data on Warning Letters Related to Dietary Supplements

Incorporating data from our prior report, figure 11 shows the number of warning letters related to dietary supplements FDA issued from January 1, 2002, through December 31, 2011. The relatively low number of letters issued in 2007 is in part due to the timing of the letters—if we calculated the number of letters issued by fiscal year, the number would be 43.

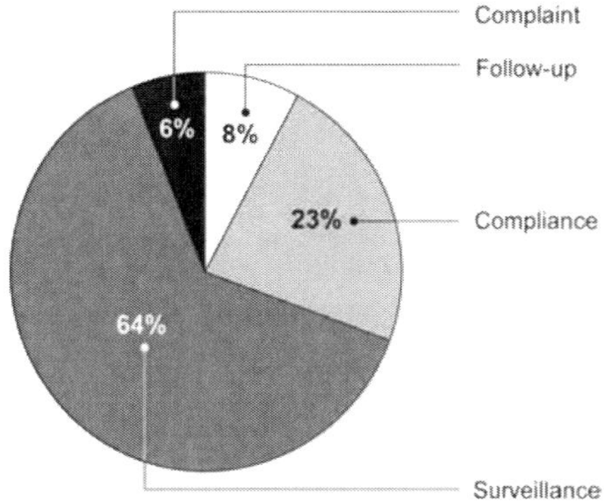

Source: GAO analysis of FDA data.

Note: Complaint inspections are conducted to investigate consumer complaints about a firm. Follow-up inspections are conducted to assess a firm's progress after an advisory or regulatory action such as a warning letter or recall. Compliance inspections are "for-cause" inspections to investigate specific compliance issues. Surveillance inspections are routine inspections that generally assess whether a firm is following dietary supplement good manufacturing practices, as applicable.

Figure 10. Type of Dietary Supplement Inspections, 2008 through 2011.

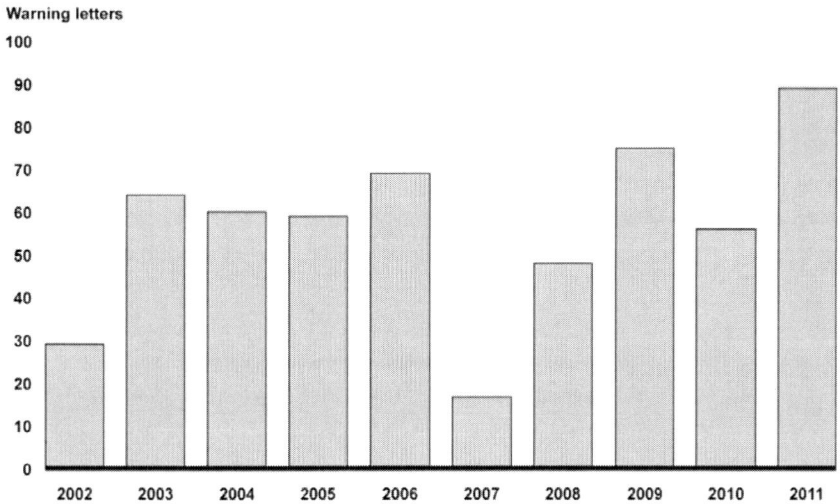

Source: GAO analysis of FDA data.

Figure 11. Number of Warning Letters Related to Dietary Supplements, 2002 through 2011.

Data on Recalls Related to Dietary Supplements

Figure 12 shows the number of Class I, health fraud, and other safety-related voluntary recalls related to dietary supplements from January 1, 2008, through December 31, 2011. We focused on these three types of recalls because FDA determined they (1) are the most likely to cause a serious health problem, (2) could cause a serious health problem, or (3) considered them to be of sufficient concern to issue a safety alert press release.

Data on Imports Related to Dietary Supplements

Figure 13 shows the number of import refusals by product type from January 1, 2008, through December 31, 2011.

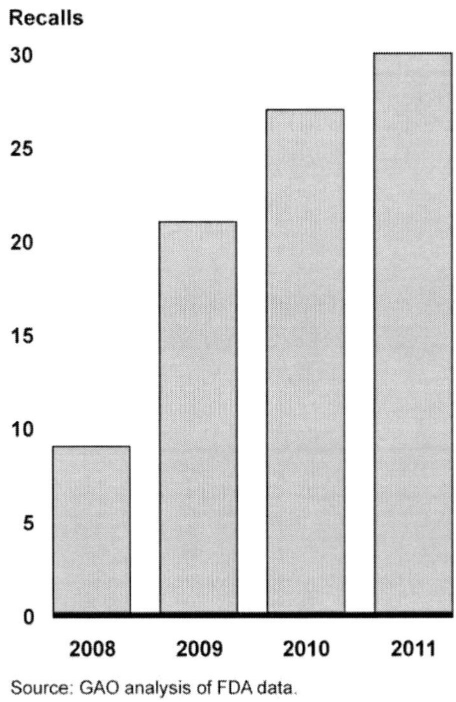

Source: GAO analysis of FDA data.

Figure 12. Number of Class I, Health Fraud, and Other Safety-Related Dietary Supplement Recalls, 2008 through 2011.

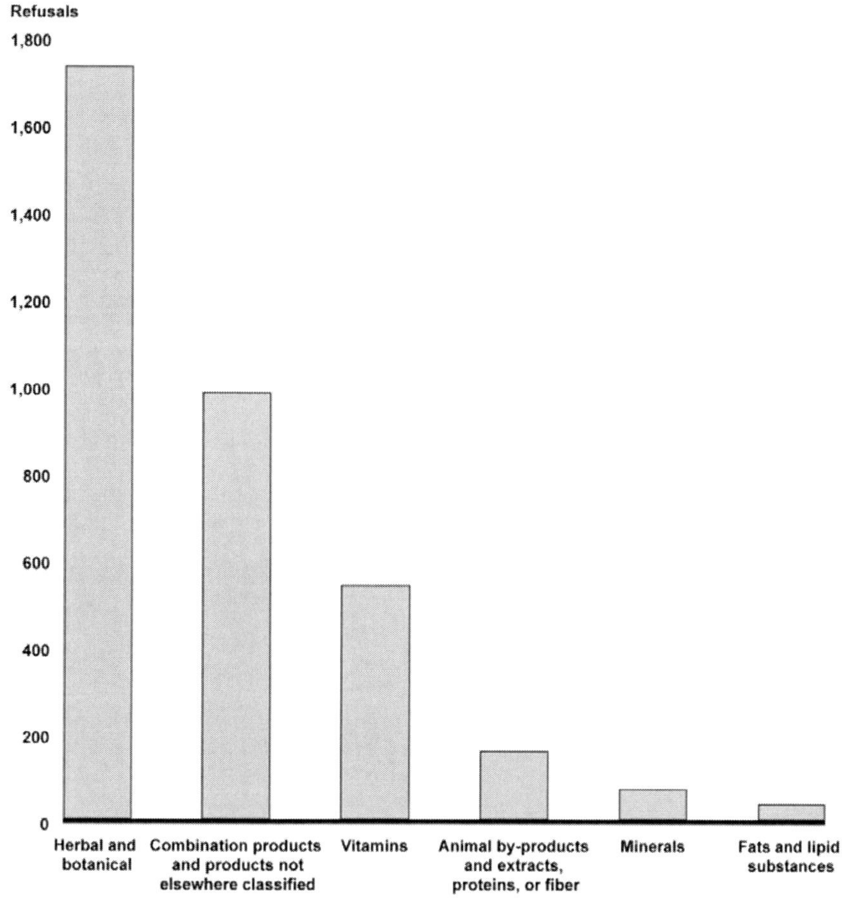

Source: GAO analysis of FDA data.

Note: To be consistent with our prior report, GAO-09-250, these data only include products classified as dietary supplements and do not include products that were initially classified as dietary supplements, then reclassified as drugs by FDA. (FDA reclassifies dietary supplements as drugs if the products contain an active pharmaceutical ingredient or if their labeling contains claims or other evidence that would cause them to be regulated as drugs.) FDA did not provide information on how many dietary supplements were reclassified as drugs and, therefore, refused entry to the United States. These data are current as of April 13, 2012.

Figure 13. Dietary Supplement Import Refusals by Product Type, 2008 through 2011.

End Notes

[1] Nutrition Business Journal, *NBJ's Supplement Business Report 2012* (Boulder, CO: Penton Media Inc: 2012) at http://newhope360.com/research/supplement-business-report (accessed December 12, 2012).

[2] According to the Dietary Supplement Health and Education Act of 1994, the estimated 600 dietary supplement manufacturers in the United States produced approximately 4,000 products, with total annual sales of such products alone reaching at least $4 billion at that time.

[3] GAO, *Dietary Supplements Containing Ephedra: Health Risks and FDA's Oversight,* GAO-03-1042T (Washington, D.C.: July 23, 2003).

[4] Products may include "proprietary blends," which must list all ingredients but do not need to list the amount of each ingredient.

[5] Although FDA does not approve dietary supplements, a dietary supplement manufacturer or distributor of a supplement with a "new dietary ingredient"—an ingredient that was not marketed in the United States before October 15, 1994—may be required to notify FDA at least 75 days before marketing the product, depending on the history of use of the ingredient.

[6] The significant risk of illness or injury standard applies under conditions of recommended or suggested use, or if no conditions are recommended or suggested, under conditions of ordinary use.

[7] Firms are required to report serious adverse events to FDA that occur on or after December 22, 2007, but since the law allows firms 15 days to file a report with FDA, the agency did not receive its first mandatory report until January 2008. Firms are also required to report follow-up medical information received about serious adverse events within 1 year after the initial report.

[8] S. Rep. No. 109-324 (2006).

[9] GAO, *Dietary Supplements: FDA Should Take Further Actions to Improve Oversight and Consumer Understanding,* GAO-09-250 (Washington, D.C.: Jan. 29, 2009).

[10] GAO, *Food Safety: Improvements Needed in Overseeing the Safety of Dietary Supplements and "Functional Foods,"* GAO/RCED-00-156 (Washington, D.C.: July 11, 2000).

[11] The Federal Food, Drug, and Cosmetic Act generally requires that when a company adds an ingredient to a food product, that ingredient must either be generally recognized as safe (GRAS) or go through FDA's review and approval process as a food additive. The GRAS standard is defined as a general recognition among qualified experts that the substance is reasonably certain to be safe under the conditions of its intended use (21 U.S.C. §§ 321(s), 348). See GAO, *FDA Should Strengthen Its Oversight of Food Ingredients Determined to Be Generally Recognized as Safe (GRAS),* GAO-10-246 (Washington, D.C.: Feb. 3, 2010) for more information.

[12] According to FDA officials, CAERs also collects data on adverse events related to cosmetics.

[13] Other responsibilities include managing reviews of regulatory actions recommended by field offices and guiding field offices' activities, when necessary, in developing scientifically and legally supportable actions.

[14] According to FDA officials, the Office of Regulatory Affairs also coordinates with FDA's Office of Chief Counsel for advisory and regulatory actions.

[15] Individuals may also call or e-mail health problems directly to CFSAN; however, CFSAN officials told us relatively few do so.

[16] Consumer complaints are not limited to health problems but may include problems with products, such as foul odors or bottles containing a pill that is different than the other pills in the container.

[17] These centers were formerly known as poison control centers. In addition to receiving calls about poison exposures where there is an identifiable exposed person, poison centers also

receive calls where there is no identifiable exposed person, which poison centers treat as information cases.

[18] Poison centers are typically affiliated with state government agencies or academic medical centers, according to American Association of Poison Control Centers (AAPCC) representatives.

[19] The AAPCC manages a 24-hour hotline that provides free medical advice from toxicology specialists including nurses, pharmacists, physicians, and poison information providers. All local poison centers can be reached through the 24-hour hotline.

[20] According to AAPCC representatives, poison centers have shared information with FDA and other public health agencies, such as the Centers for Disease Control and Prevention, when they detect potential signals of an outbreak, such as a foodborne illness, based on a pattern of calls to their centers.

[21] FDA uses product codes to classify the products it regulates. For dietary supplements, these codes contain information about the industry, the type of ingredient, the delivery mechanism (e.g., capsule, topical), and whether the product is intended for human or animal use. The general categories for types of supplement ingredients are vitamin, mineral, protein, herbal and botanical, animal byproducts and extracts, fats and lipid substances, fiber, and a category for products that either combine different types of ingredients, such as vitamins and botanicals, or are otherwise not classified into one of the other categories. A vitamin C supplement with Echinacea is an example of a combination product that would fall into this category. Royal jelly—a byproduct of honey bees—is an example of a not elsewhere classified supplement that would fall into this category.

[22] CFSAN officials noted that the program subject matter experts in the Division of Dietary Supplement Programs are medical officers.

[23] This average does not include cases where both a voluntary and a mandatory AER were submitted independently for the same adverse event. To avoid double-counting, we included these cases in our mandatory AER total.

[24] GAO-09-250.

[25] See e.g., *In re Hydroxycut Marketing and Sales Practices Litigation*, No. 09 2087 (S.D. Cal. Oct. 16, 2009).

[26] The case considered whether a plaintiff could state a claim for securities fraud under §10(b) of the Securities Exchange Act of 1934, as amended, and Securities and Exchange Commission Rule 10b-5, based on a pharmaceutical firm's not disclosing reports of adverse events and pending lawsuits associated with a product if the plaintiff did not allege statistically significant evidence linking adverse effects to the use of the product. *Matrixx Initiatives, Inc. v. Siracusano*. 563 U.S. ___, No. 09 Civ.1156. (Mar. 22, 2011).

[27] Because each AER can report multiple outcomes, numbers and percentages of outcomes should not be totaled.

[28] Specifically, under the Federal Food, Drug, and Cosmetic Act, the submission by a firm of an AER in compliance with the requirements of the statute is not to be construed as an admission that the dietary supplement involved caused or contributed to the adverse event.

[29] FDA officials told us they are in the process of standardizing product names across AER records.

[30] These numbers are approximate for the following reasons. First, product names may change over time, as firms alter their labeling without changing the underlying product. For example, a firm may decide to relabel its product line by age ranges (e.g., children, adults, seniors). Although we incorporated these changes into our analysis to the extent they were identifiable within the product names themselves, we did not conduct extensive research to verify these changes were not present otherwise. Second, FDA officials told us that their method for determining how many AERs are associated with a particular product varies depending on the purpose of the analysis. In some cases, it might be appropriate to consider products with the same active ingredients but different flavors to be the same product. In

other cases, FDA would consider products with different flavor formulations to be separate products.

[31]J.K. Glisson and L.A. Walker, "How physicians should evaluate dietary supplements," *American Journal of Medicine* 123, No. 7 (2010):577-582. M. Cellini et al., "Dietary Supplements: Physician Knowledge and Adverse Event Reporting," *Medicine and Science in Sports and Exercise,* 45, No. 1 (2013): 23-28. GAO .

[32] Department of Health and Human Services, Office of Inspector General, *Dietary Supplements: Companies May Be Difficult To Locate in an Emergency* (Washington, D.C.: Oct. 2012).

[33] Underreporting to adverse event systems is not unique to dietary supplements. In our prior work, we noted that similar problems exist for FDA's adverse event reporting system for pharmaceutical drugs. See GAO, *Drug Safety: FDA Has Begun Efforts to Enhance Postmarket Safety, but Additional Actions Are Needed,* GAO-10-68 (Washington, D.C.: Nov. 9, 2009).

[34] Poison centers do not define dietary supplements according to the Federal Food, Drug, and Cosmetic Act. Therefore, we worked with AAPCC representatives and FDA officials to make the appropriate adjustments to the data to make them comparable to FDA's AERs. For more information on our scope and methodology, see appendix I.

[35] Based on discussions with FDA officials, we focused our analysis on adverse events under use as directed, since these types of cases were most similar in nature to the types of AERs FDA received.

[36] Because FDA officials told us that AERs are primarily associated with product use as directed, we adjusted the poison center data to include only those cases where an individual experienced an adverse reaction when using the product as directed and excluded reports resulting from misuse, abuse, or accidental ingestion.

[37]AAPCC representatives said that they had offered to provide FDA with a smaller, targeted analysis of the dietary supplement data at no charge to temporarily meet FDA's needs while a longer-term agreement was negotiated, but CFSAN officials told us that they needed to see the raw data for such an analysis to be informative and prior to agreeing to a longer-term arrangement. AAPCC representatives told us that since they do not own the poison center data—only the national database where it is stored—they cannot release it without the 57 poison centers' permission.

[38] The Lewin Group, *Final Report on the Value of the Poison Center System, (*Falls Church, VA: The Lewin Group: 2012) http://production-aapcc.dotcloud.com/about/lewin-group-report/ (accessed January 7, 2013). The report notes that its findings do not include recent reductions in federal funding to poison centers. Additionally, according to AAPCC representatives, AAPCC funding and data management costs were not included in this report.

[39] National Academy of Sciences, Institute of Medicine, *Forging a Poison Prevention and Control System* (Washington, D.C.: 2004).

[40] According to the 2012 Lewin Group Report, total expenditures to maintain the poison center services nationwide were an estimated $136 million in 2011.

[41] According to AAPCC representatives, AAPCC does not own the data collected by poison centers, but owns and operates the national database where the data are stored. These representatives said that there are large costs for collecting, maintaining, analyzing, organizing and reporting on the national data which are borne by AAPCC and its members, and that the sales of the national data support these costs. As of February, 2013, the annual operating budget for the national database was approximately $3 million, according to an AAPCC representative.

[42] This number does not include resources for CAERS staff, as they perform center-wide surveillance activities and are budgeted separately. FDA officials said that there is also a concurrent negotiation effort underway at the department level to obtain access to AAPCC data for multiple HHS components, including CDC and FDA.

[43] FDA received more than 1.8 million AERs related to prescription drugs from 2008 to 2010, in comparison to the 3,827 FDA received related to dietary supplements from 2008 to 2010. Prescription drug AERs include those that are submitted directly to FDA and four types of AERs submitted to FDA by manufacturers for health problems, depending on the nature of the health problem, whether the health problem is described as a potential side effect in the product labeling, and the type of product.

[44] Wolkin et al., "Using Poison Center Data for National Public Health Surveillance for Chemical and Poison Exposure and Associated Illness," *Annals of Emergency Medicine* 59, no. 1 (2011): 56-61. Department of Health and Human Services, Office of Inspector General, *Adverse Event Reporting for Dietary Supplements: An Inadequate Safety Valve* (Washington, D.C.: April 2001).

[45] Haller et al., "Dietary Supplement Adverse Events: Report of a One-Year Poison Center Surveillance Project," *Journal of Medical Toxicology* 4, no. 2 (2008): 84-92. This paper considered active surveillance to include prompt follow-up of symptomatic cases, laboratory analysis, and a causality assessment by a case review panel. CFSAN officials said that they will contact firms and voluntary reporters to follow up on incomplete AERs, but often they are unable to obtain the missing information.

[46] According to CDC officials, CDC has also performed limited, targeted surveillance of poison center data for adverse events related to Hydroxycut™ and "Miracle Mineral Solution" products.

[47] For the purposes of this report, we requested data on inspections of firms that produce dietary supplements for human food use. FDA officials told us that they do not distinguish between firms that produce dietary supplements for human food use as opposed to dietary supplement firms that produce products that otherwise meet the statutory definition of dietary supplements but are for animal or drug uses, within their firm inventory database. Accordingly, the number of dietary supplement firms in the inspection inventory includes firms that produce such products for animal and drug uses. Consequently, the percent of dietary supplement firms for human food use represented by the inspections is presented as a minimum estimate.

[48] FDA contracts with states to conduct domestic facility inspections for foods and other regulated products. From January 1, 2008, to September 30, 2012, states conducted 35 domestic inspections of dietary supplement firms on FDA's behalf.

[49] Investigators from FDA district offices conduct inspections. For our determination for whether FDA identified a problem or concern during an inspection, we included all cases with a district decision of Official Action Indicated—OAI (A); Voluntary Action Indicated—VAI (E); and Referred to Center (P)—for dietary supplements, CFSAN—plus all cases where the investigator completed an inspectional observation form—a form used by FDA to document concerns observed during inspections. Concerns identified on the inspectional observation forms are preliminary findings and vary in severity. Each inspection was counted only once.

[50] Department of Health and Human Services, Office of Inspector General, *Dietary Supplements: Companies May Be Difficult To Locate in an Emergency* (Washington, D.C.: October 2012).

[51] According to Office of Inspector General officials, they asked FDA if retail-based product surveillance was a viable method for monitoring firms' compliance with AER requirements. According to these officials, FDA officials said that FDA would need too many staff resources to do the same type of study.

[52] For example, FDA officials said that supplements adulterated with active pharmaceutical ingredients or their analogues can become apparent through AER surveillance because of telltale symptoms associated with adverse reactions to these ingredients, such as cardiovascular issues and color blindness associated with the presence of prescription male sexual enhancement medications.

[53] In addition, of the 57 companies with registered facilities, 16 had inaccurate addresses listed in the registry. According to FDA officials, FDA identifies facilities for inspection from its Official Establishment Inventory (OEI), not the food facility registry. However, new or updated information about facilities entered into the food facility registry does inform FDA's maintenance of its OEI.

[54] The Federal Food, Drug, and Cosmetic Act establishes that a firm's submission of an AER cannot be construed as an admission that the dietary supplement product caused the adverse event.

[55] According to FDA guidance, these details are not part of the minimum data elements required for submitting a serious adverse event report.

[56] The causality determinations are based on a World Health Organization classification system. During the course of our review, FDA revisited prior reviewer evaluations for consistency—which reduced the causality determinations from: certain – 14 percent; probable – 14 percent; and possible – 35 percent. Most of these cases were moved to the insufficient information category for the final evaluations.

[57] Consumer complaints that involve health problems are entered into CAERS and sent directly to the Office of Compliance, according to FDA officials. Additionally, if a medical reviewer believes that a dietary supplement associated with an AER might be adulterated with an FDA-approved drug or its analogue, the reviewer will forward the report to FDA's Center for Drug Evaluation and Research.

[58] FDA received more than 20 reports over the 7-year period leading up to the firm's voluntary recall of Hydroxycut.™

[59] Outside of trying to establish whether or not an AER was part of the basis for taking a consumer protection action, we did not identify the individual basis for each of the roughly 4,700 consumer protection actions we reviewed.

[60] In 2001, the HHS Inspector General reported that it was able to document only 32 safety actions based on FDA's adverse event reporting system for dietary supplements between January 1994 and June 2000. According to the Inspector General, this number was strikingly low given that more than 100 million people were using dietary supplements at the time. Department of Health and Human Services, Office of Inspector General, *Adverse Event Reporting for Dietary Supplements: An Inadequate Safety Valve* (Washington, D.C.: April 2001).

[61] GAO, *Managing for Results: Enhancing Agency Use of Performance Information for Management Decision Making,* GAO-05-927 (Washington, D.C.: Sept. 9, 2005). For information on using performance data to improve IT strategic planning and investment management, see GAO-12-346 , *Information Technology: FDA Needs to Fully Implement Key Management Practices to Lessen Modernization Risks* (Washington, D.C.: Mar. 15, 2012).

[62] OMB, *Memorandum for the Heads of Executive Departments and Agencies: Open Government Directive, M-10-06* (Washington, D.C.: Dec. 8, 2009); HHS *Open Government Plan Version 2.0* (Washington, D.C.: Apr. 9, 2012); GAO, *Information Technology: OMB's Dashboard Has Increased Transparency and Oversight, but Improvements Needed,* GAO-10-701 (Washington, D.C.: July 16, 2010)*;* and GAO, *Electronic Government Act: Agencies Have Implemented Most Provisions, but Key Areas of Attention Remain,*GAO-12-782 (Washington, D.C.: Sept. 12, 2012).

[63] 21 U.S.C. § 355(k)(5).

[64] Information on AERs related to dietary supplements is found on FDA's performance measures webpage for CFSAN, under the archived version of performance measures for CFSAN's Office of Food Defense, Communication, and Emergency Response at http://www.fda.gov/AboutFDA/Transparency/track/ucm240881.htm (accessed December, 11, 2012).

[65] One such example provided by FDA officials is the "Protected Information" provision of section 761 of the Federal Food, Drug, and Cosmetic Act, as added by the 2006 act and codified at 21 U.S.C. § 379aa-1(f).

[66] Navin K. Kapur and Kiran Musunuru, "Clinical efficacy and safety of statins in managing cardiovascular risk," *Vascular Health and Risk Management* 4, no. 2 (2008): 341-353.

[67] Carlo Piccinni et al., "Assessing the association of pioglitazone use and bladder cancer through drug adverse event reporting," *Diabetes Care* 34, no. 6 (2011): 1,369-71.

[68] Elisabetta Poluzzi et al., "Antimicrobials and the risk of Torsades de Pointes: The contribution from data mining of the U.S. FDA Adverse Event Reporting System," *Drug Safety* 33, no. 4 (2010): 303-314.

[69] Increasing the amount of publicly-available information on its website about AERs for all FDA-regulated products was also the focus of a draft proposal under FDA's Transparency Initiative in May, 2010. We asked FDA officials if expanding public access to dietary supplement AERs was under consideration as part of this initiative, and they said it was not.

[70] GAO.

[71] GAO-09-250. For example, bitter orange—historically used as a flavoring—could be reformulated into a product that is 95 percent synephrine, a powerful stimulant. FDA officials said that even without guidance, firms must meet their statutory obligation to notify FDA. However, the preamble to the draft NDI guidance states that the purpose of the guidance is to assist industry in deciding when a premarket safety notification for an NDI is necessary; the chemical alteration of historical ingredients is one of the questions addressed.

[72] *Consumer Reports*, "The Buzz on Energy-Drink Caffeine" at http://www.consumerreports.org/cro/magazine/2012/12/the-buzz-on-energy-drink-caffeine/index.htm (accessed December 10, 2012); Higgins et al., "Energy Beverages: Content and Safety," *Mayo Clinic Proceedings* 85, no. 11(2010); and Substance Abuse and Mental Health Services Administration, Center for Behavioral Health Statistics and Quality, *The Dawn Report: Emergency Department Visits Involving Energy Drinks (*Rockville, MD: Nov. 22, 2011).

[73] FDA officials told us their basis for grouping products together depends on the particular analytical need. For example, in some cases, products with the same active ingredient but different flavors would be grouped similarly and, in other cases, products with different flavors would be grouped separately.

[74] *Class I* recalls involve a reasonable probability that the use of or exposure to a violative product will cause serious adverse health problems or death. *Class II* recalls involve violative products that may cause temporary or medically reversible adverse health problems or where the probability of serious adverse health problems is remote. *Class III* recalls involves violative products not likely to cause adverse health problems.

[75] We collected data on Class II and Class III recalls from FDA's Recall Enterprise System related to dietary supplements. However, we could not verify that the data were complete because of inconsistencies in how tainted supplement products are classified within the database. In some cases, they are classified as drugs, in other cases; they are classified as dietary supplements. We were able to verify the universe for Class I recalls against FDA press releases on its Recalls, Market Withdrawals, and Safety Alerts web page and Recalls - Health Fraud web page, but did not verify Class II and Class III recalls because according to FDA they are less likely to cause a serious health problem.

[76] We did not include consumer complaints in this analysis because consumer complaints with adverse events are uploaded into the CAERS database as voluntary AERs and thus the matching process would yield false positives.

[77] GAO.

In: Dietary Supplements and FDA Use … ISBN: 978-1-62808-023-0
Editor: William M. Forsberg

Chapter 2

DIETARY SUPPLEMENTS - REPORTING AN ADVERSE EVENT AT A GLANCE*

U.S. Food and Drug Administration

THE REQUIREMENT

Manufacturers, packers, and distributors of dietary supplements in the United States are required to report information about serious adverse effects associated with the use of these supplements to the Food and Drug Administration (FDA).

This requirement is detailed in the Dietary Supplement and Nonprescription Drug Consumer Protection Act, enacted on December 22, 2006. The effective date for complying with this requirement was December 22, 2007.

WHAT IS A DIETARY SUPPLEMENT?

For the purposes of reporting an adverse event to the FDA, dietary supplements are products intended to supplement the diet and include one or more of the following ingredients:

* This document was released March 2013.

- Vitamins
- Minerals
- Herbs or other botanicals
- Amino acids
- Any dietary substance for use by man to supplement the diet by increasing total dietary intake or any concentrate, metabolite, constituent, or extract or any combination of any ingredient listed above.

WHO MUST REPORT

The manufacturer, packer, or distributor of a dietary supplement marketed in the United States whose name appears on the label of the supplement is required to report serious adverse events.

According to the law, a dietary supplement label must include contact information (the domestic address or phone number) for the supplement's manufacturer, packer, or distributor. The law refers to this entity as the "responsible person."

WHAT EVENTS MUST BE REPORTED

The "responsible person" must report any serious adverse event associated with the use of dietary supplements.

An adverse event is "any health-related event associated with the use of a dietary supplement that is adverse." A serious adverse event is an adverse event that:

- Results in:
    - Death
    - A life-threatening experience
    - Inpatient hospitalization
    - A persistent or significant disability or incapacity
    - A congenital anomaly or birth defect; or
- Requires, based on a reasonable medical judgment, a medical or surgical intervention to prevent an outcome described above.

FDA is authorized to have access to all adverse event report records that dietary supplement manufacturers, packers, and distributors are required to maintain.

How to Submit an Adverse Event Report

To submit a serious adverse event report for a dietary supplement:

1. Go to Reporting Serious Problems to the FDA: Download Forms.
2. Click Form FDA 3500A – Mandatory Reporting.
3. Complete the following sections of MedWatch Form FDA 3500A:
   - Patient Information (Section A):
   - Adverse Event or Product Problems (Section B): Note that blocks 5 and 6 are not required for reports on dietary supple ments.
   - Suspect Product (Section C)
   - Initial Reporter (Section E)
   - All Manufacturers (Section G)
4. Obtain a copy of the label of the dietary supplement.
5. Mail the form along with the product label to this address:

U.S. Food and Drug Administration CAERS Team HFS-11
5100 Paint Branch Parkway
College Park, MD 20740

Note: Reports may not be submitted electronically or by fax.

Send follow-up reports with additional medical information to this same address.

For more information on completing the form, see Instructions for Completing the MedWatch Form 3500A to Report a Serious Adverse Event Associated with a Dietary Supplement.

When to Submit Reports

The following must be submitted to FDA no later than 15 business days after the report is received by the "responsible person":

- Any serious adverse event report
- All follow-up reports of new medical information.

REPORT SUBMISSION IS NOT AN ADMISSION OF FAULT

Submitting a serious adverse event report will not be construed by FDA as an admission that the dietary supplement involved caused or contributed to the adverse event being reported, or that any person included in the report caused or contributed to the event.

HOW LONG MUST ADVERSE EVENT REPORTS BE KEPT?

Adverse event reports and related records must be maintained for a period of 6 years. For each serious adverse event this includes:

- The original MedWatch Form FDA 3500A form submitted and any attachments
- Any related medical information received after submitting the initial report
- Any reports submitted to FDA including new medical information
- Communications between the "responsible person" and the initial reporter or any other person who provided information related to the adverse event.

For more information

On the *FDA.gov* website go to Food>Dietary Supplements> Guidance, Compliance, & Regulatory Information.

- The Law: Dietary Supplement and Nonprescription Drug Consumer Protection Act
- Guidance for Industry: Questions and Answers Regarding Adverse Event Reporting and Recordkeeping for Dietary Supplements
- Instructions: Completing the MedWatch Form 3500A to Report a Serious Adverse Event Associated with a Dietary Supplement

You may also email questions to CAERS@fda.hhs.gov

In: Dietary Supplements and FDA Use … ISBN: 978-1-62808-023-0
Editor: William M. Forsberg

Chapter 3

Q&A ON DIETARY SUPPLEMENTS*

U.S. Food and Drug Administration

GENERAL QUESTIONS:

- What is a dietary supplement?
- What is a "new dietary ingredient" in a dietary supplement?
- Should I check with my doctor or healthcare provider before using a supplement?
- What is FDA's role in regulating dietary supplements versus the manufacturer's responsibility for marketing them?
- When must a manufacturer or distributor notify FDA about a dietary supplement it intends to market in the U.S.?
- What information must the manufacturer disclose on the label of a dietary supplement?
- Must all ingredients be declared on the label of a dietary supplement?
- Are dietary supplement serving sizes standardized or are there restrictions on the amount of a nutrient that can be in one serving?
- Where can I get information about a specific dietary supplement?
- What are some tips on searching the Web for information on dietary supplements?

---

* This is an edited, reformatted and augmented version of the U.S. Food and Drug Administration publication, dated April 2013.

- Who has the responsibility for ensuring that a dietary supplement is safe?
- Do manufacturers or distributors of dietary supplements have to tell FDA or consumers what evidence they have about their product's safety or what evidence they have to back up the claims they are making for them?
- How can consumers inform themselves about safety and other issues related to dietary supplements?
- What is FDA's oversight responsibility for dietary supplements?
- Does FDA routinely analyze the content of dietary supplements?
- Is it legal to market a dietary supplement product as a treatment or cure for a specific disease or condition?
- Who validates claims and what kinds of claims can be made on dietary supplement labels?
- Why do some supplements have wording (a disclaimer) that says: "This statement has not been evaluated by the FDA. This product is not intended to diagnose, treat, cure, or prevent any disease"?
- How are advertisements for dietary supplements regulated?
- How do I, my health care provider, or any informed individual report a problem or illness caused by a dietary supplement to FDA?

What Is a Dietary Supplement?

Congress defined the term "dietary supplement" in the Dietary Supplement Health and Education Act (DSHEA) of 1994. A dietary supplement is a product taken by mouth that contains a "dietary ingredient" intended to supplement the diet. The "dietary ingredients" in these products may include: vitamins, minerals, herbs or other botanicals, amino acids, and substances such as enzymes, organ tissues, glandulars, and metabolites. Dietary supplements can also be extracts or concentrates, and may be found in many forms such as tablets, capsules, softgels, gelcaps, liquids, or powders. They can also be in other forms, such as a bar, but if they are, information on their label must not represent the product as a conventional food or a sole item of a meal or diet. Whatever their form may be, DSHEA places dietary supplements in a special category under the general umbrella of "foods," not drugs, and requires that every supplement be labeled a dietary supplement.

What Is a "New Dietary Ingredient" in a Dietary Supplement?

The Dietary Supplement Health and Education Act (DSHEA) of 1994 defined both of the terms "dietary ingredient" and "new dietary ingredient" as components of dietary supplements. In order for an ingredient of a dietary supplement to be a "dietary ingredient," it must be one or any combination of the following substances:

- a vitamin,
- a mineral,
- an herb or other botanical,
- an amino acid,
- a dietary substance for use by man to supplement the diet by increasing the total dietary intake (e.g., enzymes or tissues from organs or glands), or
- a concentrate, metabolite, constituent or extract.

A "new dietary ingredient" is one that meets the above definition for a "dietary ingredient" and was not sold in the U.S. in a dietary supplement before October 15, 1994.

Should I Check with My Doctor or Healthcare Provider Before Using a Supplement?

See *Tips For The Savvy Supplement User: Making Informed Decisions And Evaluating Information.*

(http://www.fda.gov/Food/DietarySupplements/UsingDietarySupplements/ucm110567.htm)

What Is FDA's Role in Regulating Dietary Supplements Versus the Manufacturer's Responsibility for Marketing Them?

In October 1994, the Dietary Supplement Health and Education Act (DSHEA) was signed into law by President Clinton. Before this time, dietary supplements were subject to the same regulatory requirements as were other foods. This new law, which amended the Federal Food, Drug, and Cosmetic

Act, created a new regulatory framework for the safety and labeling of dietary supplements.

Under DSHEA, a firm is responsible for determining that the dietary supplements it manufactures or distributes are safe and that any representations or claims made about them are substantiated by adequate evidence to show that they are not false or misleading. This means that dietary supplements do not need approval from FDA before they are marketed. Except in the case of a new dietary ingredient, where pre-market review for safety data and other information is required by law, a firm does not have to provide FDA with the evidence it relies on to substantiate safety or effectiveness before or after it markets its products.

Also, manufacturers need to register themselves pursuant to the Bioterrorism Act (http://www.fda.gov/RegulatoryInformation/ Legislation/ ucm148797.htm) with FDA before producing or selling supplements. In June, 2007, FDA published comprehensive regulations for Current Good Manufacturing Practices for those who manufacture, package or hold dietary supplement products. These regulations focus on practices that ensure the identity, purity, quality, strength and composition of dietary supplements.

When Must A Manufacturer or Distributor Notify FDA About a Dietary Supplement It Intends to Market in the U.S.?

The Dietary Supplement Health and Education Act (DSHEA) requires that a manufacturer or distributor notify FDA if it intends to market a dietary supplement in the U.S. that contains a "new dietary ingredient." The manufacturer (and distributor) must demonstrate to FDA why the ingredient is reasonably expected to be safe for use in a dietary supplement, unless it has been recognized as a food substance and is present in the food supply.

There is no authoritative list of dietary ingredients that were marketed before October 15, 1994. Therefore, manufacturers and distributors are responsible for determining if a dietary ingredient is "new", and if it is not, for documenting that the dietary supplements its sells, containing the dietary ingredient, were marketed before October 15, 1994. For more detailed information, see *new dietary ingredients* (http://www.fda.gov/Food/Dietary Supplements/NewDietaryIngredientsNotificationProcess/ucm109764.htm).

What Information Must the Manufacturer Disclose on the Label of a Dietary Supplement?

FDA regulations require that certain information appear on dietary supplement labels. Information that must be on a dietary supplement label includes: a descriptive name of the product stating that it is a "supplement;" the name and place of business of the manufacturer, packer, or distributor; a complete list of ingredients; and the net contents of the product.

In addition, each dietary supplement (except for some small volume products or those produced by eligible small businesses) must have nutrition labeling in the form of a "Supplement Facts" panel. This label must identify each dietary ingredient contained in the product.

Must All Ingredients Be Declared on the Label of a Dietary Supplement?

Yes, ingredients not listed on the "Supplement Facts" panel must be listed in the "other ingredient" statement beneath the panel. The types of ingredients listed there could include the source of dietary ingredients, if not identified in the "Supplement Facts" panel (e.g., rose hips as the source of vitamin C), other food ingredients (e.g., water and sugar), and technical additives or processing aids (e.g., gelatin, starch, colors, stabilizers, preservatives, and flavors). For more details, see: Federal Register Final Rule - 62 FR 49826 September 23, 1997.

Are Dietary Supplement Serving Sizes Standardized or Are There Restrictions on the Amount of a Nutrient That Can Be in One Serving?

Other than the manufacturer's responsibility to ensure safety, there are no rules that limit a serving size or the amount of a nutrient in any form of dietary supplements.

This decision is made by the manufacturer and does not require FDA review or approval.

Where Can I Get Information About a Specific Dietary Supplement?

Manufacturers and distributors do not need FDA approval to sell their dietary supplements. This means that FDA does not keep a list of manufacturers, distributors or the dietary supplement products they sell. If you want more detailed information than the label tells you about a specific product, you may contact the manufacturer of that brand directly. The name and address of the manufacturer or distributor can be found on the label of the dietary supplement.

What Are Some Tips on Searching the Web for Information on Dietary Supplements?

See Tips For The Savvy Supplement User: Making Informed Decisions And Evaluating Information. (http://www.fda.gov/Food/DietarySupplements/UsingDietarySupplements/ucm110567.htm)

Who Has The Responsibility for Ensuring That a Dietary Supplement Is Safe?

By law (DSHEA), the manufacturer is responsible for ensuring that its dietary supplement products are safe before they are marketed. Unlike drug products that must be proven safe and effective for their intended use before marketing, there are no provisions in the law for FDA to "approve" dietary supplements for safety or effectiveness before they reach the consumer. Under DSHEA, once the product is marketed, FDA has the responsibility for showing that a dietary supplement is "unsafe," before it can take action to restrict the product's use or removal from the marketplace. However, manufacturers and distributors of dietary supplements must record, investigate and forward to FDA any reports they receive of serious adverse events associated with the use of their products that are reported to them directly. FDA is able to evaluate these reports and any other adverse event information reported directly to us by healthcare providers or consumers to identify early signals that a product may present safety risks to consumers. You can find more information on reporting adverse events associated with the use of dietary supplements at *Dietary Supplements - Adverse Event Reporting* (http://www.fda.gov/Food/DietarySupplements/ReportAdverseEvent/ucm111110.htm).

Do Manufacturers or Distributors of Dietary Supplements Have to Tell FDA or Consumers What Evidence They Have About Their Product's Safety or What Evidence They Have to Back up the Claims They Are Making for Them?

No, except for rules described above that govern "new dietary ingredients," there is no provision under any law or regulation that FDA enforces that requires a firm to disclose to FDA or consumers the information they have about the safety or purported benefits of their dietary supplement products. Likewise, there is no prohibition against them making this information available either to FDA or to their customers. It is up to each firm to set its own policy on disclosure of such information. For more information, see *claims that can be made for dietary supplements* (http://www.fda.gov/Food/IngredientsPackagingLabeling/LabelingNutrition/ucm111447.htm)

How Can Consumers Inform Themselves About Safety and Other Issues Rel

It is important to be well informed about products before purchasing them. Because it is often difficult to know what information is reliable and what is questionable, consumers may first want to contact the manufacturer about the product they intend to purchase (see previous question "Where can I get information about a specific dietary supplement?"). In addition, to help consumers in their search to be better informed, FDA is providing the following sites: *Tips For The Savvy Supplement User: Making Informed Decisions And Evaluating Information* (http://www.fda.gov/Food/DietarySupplements/UsingDietarySupplements/ucm110567.htm)includes information on how to evaluate research findings and health information on-line and *Claims That Can Be Made for Conventional Foods and Dietary Supplements* (http://www.fda.gov/Food/IngredientsPackagingLabeling/LabelingNutrition/ucm111447.htm), provides information on what types of claims can be made for dietary supplements.

What Is FDA's Oversight Responsibility for Dietary Supplements?

Because dietary supplements are under the "umbrella" of foods, FDA's Center for Food Safety and Applied Nutrition (CFSAN) is responsible for the agency's oversight of these products. FDA's efforts to monitor the marketplace for potential *illegal* products (that is, products that may be unsafe or make false or misleading claims) include obtaining information from inspections of dietary supplement manufacturers and distributors, the Internet, consumer and trade complaints, occasional laboratory analyses of selected products, and adverse events associated with the use of supplements that are reported to the agency.

Does FDA Routinely Analyze the Content of Dietary Supplements?

In that FDA has limited resources to analyze the composition of food products, including dietary supplements, it focuses these resources first on public health emergencies and products that may have caused injury or illness. Enforcement priorities then go to products thought to be unsafe or fraudulent or in violation of the law. The remaining funds are used for routine monitoring of products pulled from store shelves or collected during inspections of manufacturing firms. The agency does not analyze dietary supplements before they are sold to consumers. The manufacturer is responsible for ensuring that the "Supplement Facts" label and ingredient list are accurate, that the dietary ingredients are safe, and that the content matches the amount declared on the label. FDA does not have resources to analyze dietary supplements sent to the agency by consumers who want to know their content. Instead, consumers may contact the manufacturer or a commercial laboratory for an analysis of the content.

Is It Legal to Market a Dietary Supplement Product as a Treatment or Cure for a Specific Disease or Condition?

No, a product sold as a dietary supplement and promoted on its label or in labeling* as a treatment, prevention or cure for a specific disease or condition would be considered an unapproved--and thus illegal--drug. To maintain the product's status as a dietary supplement, the label and labeling must be consistent with the provisions in the Dietary Supplement Health and Education Act (DSHEA) of 1994.

*Labeling refers to the label as well as accompanying material that is used by a manufacturer to promote and market a specific product.

Who Validates Claims and What Kinds of Claims Can Be Made on Dietary Supplement Labels?

FDA receives many consumer inquiries about the validity of claims for dietary supplements, including product labels, advertisements, media, and printed materials. The responsibility for ensuring the validity of these claims rests with the manufacturer, FDA, and, in the case of advertising, with the Federal Trade Commission.

By law, manufacturers may make three types of claims for their dietary supplement products: health claims, structure/function claims, and nutrient content claims. Some of these claims describe: the link between a food substance and disease or a health-related condition; the intended benefits of using the product; or the amount of a nutrient or dietary substance in a product. Different requirements generally apply to each type of claim, and are *described in more detail* (http://www.fda.gov/Food/Ingredients Packaging Labeling/LabelingNutrition/ucm111447.htm).

Why Do Some Supplements Have Wording (A Disclaimer) That Says: "This Statement Has Not Been Evaluated by the FDA. This Product is Not Intended to Diagnose, Treat, Cure, or Prevent Any Disease"?

This statement or "disclaimer" is required by law (DSHEA) when a manufacturer makes a structure/function claim on a dietary supplement label. In general, these claims describe the role of a nutrient or dietary ingredient intended to affect the structure or function of the body. The manufacturer is responsible for ensuring the accuracy and truthfulness of these claims; they are not approved by FDA. For this reason, the law says that if a dietary supplement label includes such a claim, it must state in a "disclaimer" that FDA has not evaluated this claim. The disclaimer must also state that this product is not intended to "diagnose, treat, cure or prevent any disease," because only a drug can legally make such a claim.

How Are Advertisements for Dietary Supplements Regulated?

The Federal Trade Commission (FTC) regulates advertising, including infomercials, for dietary supplements and most other products sold to consumers. FDA works closely with FTC in this area, but FTC's work is directed by different laws. For more information on FTC, go to the *FTC web site* (http://www.ftc.gov/bcp/). Advertising and promotional material received in the mail are also regulated under different laws and are subject to regulation by the U.S. Postal Inspection Service.

How Do I, My Health Care Provider, or Any Informed Individual Report a Problem or Illness Caused by a Dietary Supplement to FDA?

If you think you have suffered a serious harmful effect or illness from a product FDA regulates, including dietary supplements, the first thing you should do is contact or see your healthcare provider immediately. Then, you and your health care provider are encouraged to report this problem to FDA.

Your health care provider can call FDA's MedWatch hotline at 1-800-FDA-1088, submit a report by fax to 1-800-FDA-0178 or *on-line* (http://www.fda.gov/Safety/MedWatch/HowToReport/ucm085568.htm). The MedWatch program provides a way for health care providers to report problems believed to be caused by FDA-regulated products such as drugs, medical devices, medical foods and dietary supplements.

You, or anyone, may report a serious adverse event or illness directly to FDA if you believe it is related to the use of any of the above-mentioned products, by calling FDA at 1-800-FDA-1088, by fax at 1-800-FDA-0178 or *reporting on-line* (http://www.fda.gov/Safety/MedWatch/HowToReport/ucm053074.htm). FDA would like to know when you think a product caused you a serious problem, even if you are not sure that the product was the cause, or even if you do not visit a doctor or clinic. In addition to communicating with FDA on-line or by phone, you may use the postage-paid MedWatch form available from the FDA Web site.

NOTE: The identity of the reporter and/or patient is kept confidential.

For a general, not serious, complaint or concern about food products, including dietary supplements, you may contact the consumer complaint coordinator at the local FDA District Office nearest you. See the following Web address for the telephone number: *Consumer Complaint Coordinators* (http://www.fda.gov/Safety/ReportaProblem/ConsumerComplaintCoordinators/default.htm).

(Original website for this document (updated and viewed, April 2013) http://www.fda.gov/Food/DietarySupplements/QADietarySupplements/default.htm)

In: Dietary Supplements and FDA Use ...
Editor: William M. Forsberg
ISBN: 978-1-62808-023-0

Chapter 4

THE PUBLIC'S STAKE IN ADVERSE EVENT REPORTING*

U.S. Food and Drug Administration

The FDA carefully considers all the available safety information submitted to the agency before a product is approved. However, unexpected and sometimes serious safety problems can emerge once a product goes to market and is used by millions of people.

As a result, postmarket safety monitoring, that is, analyzing information on products once they go to market, is a critical part of the FDA's responsibilities.

The public provides an important source of such safety information. Health care facilities, practitioners, and patients submit reports to the FDA and to manufacturers on adverse events, medical errors, and product quality problems observed during the use of a product. Reporting by facilities, practitioners and patients to the FDA or to manufacturers – known either as voluntary reporting when involving medical devices and spontaneous reporting when involving drugs and biologic products – is entirely voluntary and has increased greatly in recent years. In addition to voluntary reporting, there is mandatory reporting. Manufacturers who receive a report must submit it to the FDA and healthcare facilities must file reports of deaths and serious injuries involving medical devices.

---

* This is an edited, reformatted and augmented version of the U.S. Food and Drug Administration publication, dated April 2013.

Reports to the FDA are sent to the agency's MedWatch program or to the Vaccine Adverse Event Reporting System for vaccines. MedWatch also provides an Internet gateway for finding safety information about products.

The FDA analyzes both voluntary and mandatory reports to develop hypotheses about possible adverse events. In many cases it is hard to know whether an adverse event that happens after taking a drug was caused by the medication itself because many adverse events such as stroke or heart attack can occur from other causes, such as a patient's underlying illness. But where the adverse event is very uncommon and unanticipated and the event occurs soon after the drug is started, there may be good reason to think the drug caused the adverse event.

Sometimes there is a need to conduct new studies to determine whether or not an adverse event associated with the use of a medical product was in fact caused by that product. The spontaneous reporting system is still the principal mechanism by which signals of such rare, but serious, adverse events are currently detected.

The results can be powerful: Reports of severe and in many cases fatal liver injuries resulted in the market removal of the nonsteroidal anti-inflammatory drug Duract (bromfenac) in 1998 only months after its approval. Similarly, the FDA received four reports of a serious condition affecting the bone marrow within four months after the antibiotic Zyvox (linezolid) was approved for marketing in 2000. The label was revised to inform providers about the risk for this adverse reaction and with recommendations for monitoring patients.

Safety reports about devices are also helpful. Just one report that a patient had become paralyzed following surgery on a cracked rib resulted in an important labeling change for a product used to stop bleeding where the rib connected to the spinal column. It turned out that the product could swell and put pressure on surrounding tissue, damaging the spinal cord.

Physicians at four different institutions across the United States informed the FDA about an increasing number of severe and life-threatening complications associated with metallic stents used to prop open the trachea. In response, the FDA sent out an alert to other health care practitioners. The alert warned about the risk of this complication in patients with a certain type of breathing disorder.

The bottom line: voluntary and mandatory reporting plays an important role in the FDA's postmarket safety monitoring.

(Original website for this information (viewed April 2013) http://www.fda.gov/Drugs/GuidanceComplianceRegulatoryInformation/Surveillance/AdverseDrugEffects/ucm179586.htm)

INDEX

G

H

I

J

L

M

N

O

P

Q

R